I0503405

AN EXAMINATION

OF

WEISMANNISM

BY

GEORGE JOHN ROMANES

M.A., LL.D., F.R.S.

HONORARY FELLOW OF GONVILLE AND CAIUS COLLEGE,
CAMBRIDGE

PREFACE

As already stated in the Preface to the second edition of *Darwin and after Darwin*, Part I, severe and protracted illness has hitherto prevented me from proceeding to the publication of Part II. It is now more than a year since I had to suspend work of every kind, and therefore, although at that time Part II was almost ready for press, I have not yet been able to write its concluding chapters. Shortly before and during this interval Professor Weismann has produced his essays on *Amphimixis* and *The Germ-plasm*. These works present extensive additions to, and considerable modifications of, his previous theories as collected together in the English translation, under the title *Essays on Heredity, Vol. I*. Consequently, it has become necessary for me either to re-write the examination of his system which I had prepared for Part II of my own treatise, or else to leave that examination as it stood, and to add a further chapter dealing with those later developments of his system to which I have just alluded. After due reflection I have decided upon the latter course, because in this way we are most likely to obtain a clear view of the growth of Weismann's elaborate structure of theories—a view which it is almost necessary, for the purposes of criticism, that we should obtain.

Having decided upon this point, it occurred to me that certain advantages would be gained by removing the whole criticism from the position which it was originally intended to occupy as a section of my forthcoming volume on the Post-Darwinian period. For, in consequence of the criticism having been written at successive intervals during the last six or eight years as Professor Weismann's works successively appeared, it has now swelled to a bulk which would unduly encumber the volume just mentioned. Again, the growth of Professor Weismann's system has of late become so rapid, that if the criticism is to keep pace with it in future, the best plan will doubtless be the one which it is now my intention to adopt—viz., to publish the criticism in a separate form, and in comparatively small editions, so that further chapters may be added with as much celerity as Professor Weismann may hereafter produce his successive works. Lastly, where so much elaborate speculation and so many changes of doctrine are concerned, it is inevitable that some misunderstandings on the part of a critic are likely to have arisen; and therefore, should Professor Weismann deem it worth his while to correct any such failings on my part, the plan of publication just alluded to will furnish me with the best opportunity of dealing with whatever he may have to say.

It must be understood, however, that under the term "Weismannism" I do not include any reference to the important question with which the name of Weismann has been mainly associated—i.e., the inheritance or non-inheritance of acquired characters. This is a question of fact, which stands to be answered by the inductive methods of observation and experiment: not by the deductive methods of general reasoning. Of course Professor Weismann is fully entitled to assume a negative answer as a basis whereon to construct his theory of the continuity of germ-plasm; but no amount of speculation as to what the mechanism of heredity is likely to be if once this assumption is granted, can even so much as tend to prove that the assumption itself is true. Therefore, in this "examination of Weismannism" I intend to restrict our attention to the elaborate system of theories which Weismann has reared upon his fundamental postulate of the non-inheritance of acquired characters, reserving for my next volume our consideration of this postulate itself.

Lest, however, it should be felt that "an examination of Weismannism" in which the question of the transmission of acquired characters is omitted must indeed prove a case of Hamlet without the Prince of Denmark, I may be allowed to make two observations. In the first place, this great question of fact is clearly quite distinct from that of any theories which may be framed upon either side of it. And, in the second place, the question was not raised by Weismann. It appears, indeed, from what he says, that he never caught a glimpse of it till about ten years ago, and that he then did so as a result of his own independent thought. Moreover, it is perfectly true that to him belongs the great merit of having been the first to call general attention to the subject, and so to arouse a world-wide interest with reference to it. But to suppose that the question was first propounded by Weismann is merely to display a want of acquaintance with the course of Darwinian thought in this country. As far back as 1874 I had long conversations with Darwin himself upon the matter, and under his guidance performed what I suppose are the only systematic experiments which have ever been undertaken with regard to it. These occupied more than five years of almost exclusive devotion; but, as they all proved failures, they were never published. Therefore I here mention them merely for the purpose of showing that the idea of what is now called a "continuity of germ-plasm" was present to Darwin's mind as a logically possible alternative to the one which he adopted in his theory of pangenesis—an alternative, therefore, which he was anxious to exclude by way of experimental disproof. If it be said that no one could have been aware of this in the absence of publication, I reply that I think it may be perceived by any one who reads attentively his chapter on Pangenesis. Moreover, early in the seventies his cousin, Mr. Francis Galton, published a "Theory of Heredity," which, as we shall see in the course of the following pages, presented as distinctly as could possibly be presented the question of the transmission of acquired characters, and answered it in almost exactly the same manner as Weismann did about ten years later. Lastly, as Weismann has himself been careful to point out, he was likewise anticipated in this matter by Jäger (1878), and Nussbaum and Rauber (1880).

For these reasons, then, I exclude this question from the following examination of what I think we ought to understand as distinctively "Weismannism."

G. J. R.

CHRIST CHURCH, OXFORD,
July, 1893.

CONTENTS

AN EXAMINATION OF WEISMANNISM

CHAPTER I.

SEEING that Professor Weismann's theory of heredity, besides being somewhat elaborate in itself, is presented in a series of disconnected essays, originally published at different times, it is a matter of no small difficulty to gather from the present collection of them a complete view of the system as a whole. Therefore I propose to give a brief sketch of his several cognate theories, arranged in a manner calculated to show their logical connexion one with another. And, in order also to show the relation in which his resulting theory of heredity stands to what has hitherto been the more usual way of regarding the facts, I will begin by furnishing a similarly condensed account of Mr. Darwin's theory upon the subject. It will be observed that these two theories constitute the logical extremes of explanatory thought; and therefore it may be said, in a general way, that all other modern theories of heredity—such as those of Spencer, Häckel, Elsberg, Galton, Nägeli, His, Brooks, Hertwig, and De Vries—occupy positions more or less intermediate between these two extremes. Therefore, also, we need not wait to consider these intermediate theories[2].

"When closely analyzed, Mr. Darwin's theory—or the "provisional hypothesis of Pangenesis"—will be found to embody altogether seven assumptions, namely:—

1. That all the component cells of a multicellular organism throw off inconceivably minute germs, or "gemmules," which are then dispersed throughout the whole system.

2. That these gemmules, when so dispersed and supplied with proper nutriment, multiply by self-division, and, under suitable conditions, are capable of developing into physiological cells like those from which they were originally and severally derived.

3. That, while still in this gemmular condition, these cell-seeds have for one another a mutual affinity, which leads to their being collected from all parts of the system by the reproductive glands of the organism; and that, when so collected, they go to constitute the essential material of the sexual elements—ova and spermatozoa being thus aggregated packets of gemmules, which have emanated from all the cells of all the tissues of the organism.

4. That the development of a new organism, out of the fusion of two such packets of gemmules, is due to a summation of all the developments of some of the gemmules which these two packets contain.

5. That a large proportional number of the gemmules in each packet, however, fail to develop, and are then transmitted in a dormant state to future generations, in any of which they may be developed subsequently—thus giving rise to the phenomena of reversion or atavism.

6. That in all cases the development of gemmules into the form of their parent cells depends on their suitable union with other partially developed gemmules, which precede them in the regular course of growth.

7. That gemmules are thrown off by all physiological cells, not only during the adult state of the organism, but during all stages of its development. Or, in other words, that the production of these cell-seeds depends upon the adult condition of parent cells: not upon that of the multicellular organism as a whole.

At first sight it may well appear that we have here a very formidable array of assumptions. But Darwin ably argues in favour of each of them by pointing to well-known analogies, drawn from the vital processes of living cells both in the protozoa and metazoa. For example, it is already a well-recognized doctrine of physiology that each cell of a metazoon, or multicellular organism, though to a large extent dependent on others, is likewise to a certain extent independent or autonomous, and has the power of multiplying by self-division. Therefore, as it is certain that the sexual elements (and also buds of all descriptions) include formative material of some kind, the first assumption—or that which supposes such formative matter to be participate—is certainly not a gratuitous assumption.

Again, the second assumption—viz., that this particulate and formative material is dispersed throughout all the tissues of the organism—is sustained by the fact that, both in certain plants and in certain invertebrated animals, a severed portion of the organism will develop into an entire organism similar to that from which it was derived, as, for example, is the case with a leaf of Begonia, and with portions cut from certain invertebrated animals, such as sea-anemones, jelly-fish, &c. This well-known fact in itself seems enough to prove that the formative material in question must certainly admit, at all events in many cases, of being distributed throughout all the tissues of living organisms.

The third assumption—or that which supposes the formative material to be especially aggregated in the sexual elements—is not so much an assumption as a statement of obvious fact; while the fourth, fifth, sixth, and seventh assumptions all follow deductively from their predecessors. In other words, if the first and second assumptions be granted, and if the theory is to comprise all the facts of heredity, then the remaining five assumptions are bound to follow.

To the probable objection that the supposed gemmules must be of a size impossibly minute—seeing that thousands of millions of them would have to be packed into a single ovum or spermatozoon—Darwin opposes a calculation that a cube of glass or water, having only one ten-thousandth of an inch to a side, contains somewhere between sixteen and a hundred and thirty-one billions of molecules. Again, as touching the supposed power of multiplication on the part of his gemmules, he alludes to the fact that infectious material of all kinds exhibits a ratio of increase quite as great as any that his theory requires to attribute to gemmules. Furthermore, with respect to the elective affinity of gemmules, he remarks that "in all ordinary cases of sexual reproduction, the male and female elements certainly have an elective affinity for each other": of the ten thousand species of *Compositae*, for example, "there can be no doubt that if the pollen of all these species could be simultaneously placed on the stigma of any one species, this one would elect, with unerring certainty, its own pollen."

Such, in brief outline, is Mr. Darwin's theory of Pangenesis.

Professor Weismann's theory of Germ-plasm is fundamentally based upon the great distinction, in respect of their transmissibility, between characters that are congenital and characters that are acquired. By a congenital character is meant any individual peculiarity, whether structural or mental, with which the individual is born. By an acquired character is meant any peculiarity which the individual may subsequently develop in consequence of its own individual experience. For example, a man may be born with some malformation of one of his fingers; or he may subsequently acquire such a malformation as the result of accident or disease. Now, in the former case—i.e., in that where the malformation is congenital—it is extremely probable that the peculiarity will be transmitted to his children; while in the latter case—i.e., where the malformation is subsequently acquired—it is virtually certain that it will not be transmitted to his children. And this great difference between the transmissibility of characters that are congenital and characters that are acquired extends universally as a general law throughout the vegetable as well as the animal kingdom, and in the province of mental as in that of bodily organization. Of course this general law has always been well known, and more or less fully recognized by all modern physiologists and medical men. But before the subject was taken up by Professor Weismann, it was generally supposed that the difference in question was one of degree, not one of kind. In other words, it was assumed that acquired characters, although not so fully—and therefore not so certainly— inherited as congenital characters, nevertheless were inherited in some lesser degree; so that if the same character continued to be developed successively in a number of sequent generations, what was at first only a slight tendency to be inherited would become by summation a more and more pronounced tendency, till eventually the acquired character might be as strongly inherited as any other character which was *ab initio* congenital. Now it is the validity of this assumption that is challenged by Professor Weismann. He says there is no evidence of any acquired characters being in any degree inherited; and, therefore, that in this important respect they may be held to differ from congenital characters in kind. On the supposition that they do thus differ in kind, he furnishes a very attractive theory of heredity, which serves at once to explain the difference, and to represent it as a matter of physiological impossibility that any acquired character can, under any circumstances whatsoever, be transmitted to progeny.

But, in order fully to comprehend this theory, it is desirable first of all to explain Professor Weismann's views upon certain other topics which are intimately connected with—and, indeed, logically sequent upon—the use to which he puts the distinction just mentioned.

Starting from the fact that unicellular organisms multiply by fission and gemmation, he argues that, aboriginally and potentially, life is immortal. For when a protozoon divides itself into two more or less equal parts by fission, and each of the two halves thereupon grows into another protozoon, it does not appear that there has been any death on the part of the living material involved; and inasmuch as this process of fission goes on continuously from generation to generation, there is seemingly never any death on the part of such protoplasmic material, although there is a continuous addition to it as the numbers of individuals increase. Similarly, in the case of gemmation, when a protozoon parts with a small portion of its living material in the form of a bud, this portion does not die, but develops into a new individual; and, therefore, the process is exactly analogous to that of fission, save that a small instead of a large part of the parent substance is involved. Now, if life be thus immortal in the case of unicellular organisms, why should it have ceased to be so in the case of multicellular? Weismann's answer is, that all the multicellular organisms propagate themselves, not exclusively by fission or gemmation, but by sexual fertilization, where the condition to a new organism arising is that minute and specialized portions of two parent organisms should fuse together. Now, it is evident that with this change in the method of propagation, serious disadvantage would accrue to any species if its sexual individuals were to continue to be immortal; for in that case every species which multiplies by sexual methods would in time become composed of individuals broken down and decrepit through the results of accident and disease—always operating and ever accumulating throughout the course of their immortal lives. Consequently, as soon as sexual methods of propagation superseded the more primitive a-sexual methods, it became desirable in the interests of the sexually-propagating species that their constituent individuals should cease to be immortal, so that the species should always be recuperated by fresh, young, and well-formed representatives. Consequently, also, natural selection would speedily see to it that all sexually-propagating species should become deprived of the aboriginal endowment of immortality, with the result that death is now universal among all the individuals of such species—that is to say, among all the metazoa and metaphyta. Nevertheless, it is to be remembered that this destiny extends only to the parts of the individual other than the contents of those specialized cells which constitute the reproductive elements. For although in each individual metazoon or metaphyton an innumerable number of these specialized cells are destined to perish during the life, or with the death, of the organism to which they belong, this is only due to the accident, so to speak, of their contents not having met with their complements in the opposite sex: it does not belong to their essential nature that they should perish, seeing that those which do happen to meet with their complements in the opposite sex help to form a new living individual, and so on through successive generations *ad infinitum*. Therefore the reproductive elements of the metazoa and metaphyta are in this respect precisely analogous to the protozoa: potentially, or in their own nature, they are immortal; and, like the protozoa, if they die, their death is an accident due to unfavourable circumstances. But the case is quite different with all the other parts of a multicellular organism. Here, no matter how favourable the circumstances may be, every cell contains within itself, or in its very nature, the eventual doom of death. Thus, of the metazoa and metaphyta it is the "germ-plasms" alone that retain their primitive endowment of everlasting life, passed on continuously through generation after generation of successively perishing organisms.

So far, it is contended, we are dealing with matters of fact. It must be taken as true that the protoplasm of the unicellular organisms, and the germ-plasm of the multicellular organisms, has been continuous through the time since life first appeared upon this earth; and although large quantities of each are perpetually dying through being exposed to conditions unfavourable to life, this, as Weismann presents the matter, is quite a different case from that of all the other constituent parts of multicellular organisms, which contain within themselves the doom of death. Furthermore, it appears extremely probable that this doom of death has been brought about by natural selection for the reasons assigned by Weismann—namely, because it is for the benefit of all species which perpetuate themselves by sexual methods, that their constituent individuals should not live longer than is necessary for the sake of originating the next generation, and fairly starting it in its own struggle for existence. For Weismann has shown, by a somewhat laborious though still largely imperfect research, that there is throughout all the metazoa a general correlation between the natural lifetime of individuals composing any given species and the age at which they reach maturity, or first become capable of procreation. This general correlation, however, is somewhat modified by the time during which progeny are dependent upon their parents for support and protection. Nevertheless, it is evident that this fact tends rather to confirm the view that expectation of life on the part of individuals has in all cases been determined with strict reference to the requirements of propagation, if under propagation we include the rearing as well as the production of offspring. I may observe in passing that I do not think this general law can be found to apply to plants in nearly so close a manner as Weismann has shown it to apply to animals; but, leaving this consideration aside, I think that Weismann has made out a good case in favour of such a general law with regard to animals[3].

We have come, then, to these results. Protoplasm was originally immortal, barring accidents; and it still continues to be immortal in the case of unicellular organisms which propagate a-sexually. But in the case of all multicellular organisms, which propagate sexually, natural selection has reduced the term of life within the smallest limits that in each given case are compatible with the performance of the sexual act and the subsequent rearing of progeny—reserving, however, the original endowment of immortality for the germinal elements, whereby a *continuum* of life has been secured from the earliest appearance of life until the present day.

Now, in view of these results the question arises,—Why should the sexual methods of propagation have become so general, if their effect has been that of determining the necessary death of all individuals presenting them? Why, in the course of organic evolution, should these newer methods have been imposed on all the higher organisms, when the consequence is that all these higher organisms must pay for the innovation with their lives? Weismann's answer to this question is as interesting and ingenious as all that has gone before. Seeing that sexual propagation is so general as to be practically universal among multicellular organisms, it is obvious that in some way or another it must have had a most important part to play in the general scheme of organic evolution. What, then, is the part that it does play? What is its *raison d'être*? Briefly, according to Weismann, its function is that of furnishing congenital variations to the ever-watchful agency of natural selection, in order that natural selection may always preserve the most favourable, and pass them on to the next generation by heredity. That sexual propagation is well calculated to furnish congenital variations may easily be rendered apparent. We have only to remember that at each union there is a mixture of two sets of germinal elements; that each of these was in turn the product of two other sets in the preceding generation, and so backwards *ad infinitum* in an ever doubling ratio. Remembering this, it follows that the germinal elements of no one member of a species can ever be the same as those of any other member born of different parents; on the contrary, while both are enormously complex products, each has had a different ancestral history, such that while one presents the congenital admixtures of thousands of individuals in one line of descent, the other presents similar admixtures of thousands of other individuals in a different line of descent. Consequently, when in any sexual union two of these enormously complex germinal elements fuse together, and constitute a new individual out of their joint endowments, it is perfectly certain that that individual cannot be exactly like any other individual of the same species which has been born of different parents. The chances must be infinity to one against any single mass of germ-plasm being exactly like any other mass of germ-plasm; while any amount of latitude as to difference is allowed, up to the point at which the difference becomes too pronounced to satisfy the conditions of fertilization—in which case, of course, no new individual is born. Hence, theoretically, we have here a sufficient cause for all individual variations of a congenital kind that can possibly occur within the limits of fertility, and, therefore, that can ever become actual in living organisms. In point of fact, Weismann believes—or, at any rate, provisionally maintains—that this is the sole and only cause of variations that are congenital, and therefore (according to his views) transmissible by heredity. Now, whether or not he is right as regards these latter points, I think there can be no question that sexual propagation is, at all events, one of the main causes of congenital variation; and seeing of what enormous importance congenital variation must always have been in supplying material for the operation of natural selection, we appear to have found a most satisfactory answer to our question,—Why has sexual propagation become so universal among all the higher plants and animals? It has become so because it is thus shown to have been the condition to producing congenital variations, which in turn constitute one of the primary conditions to the working of natural selection.

Having got thus far, I should like to make two or three subsidiary remarks. In the first place, it ought to be observed that this theory touching the causes of congenital variations was not originally propounded by Professor Weismann, but occurs in the writings of several previous authors, and is expressly alluded to by Darwin[4]. Nevertheless, it occupies so prominent a place in Weismann's system of theories, and has by him been wrought up so much more elaborately than by any of his predecessors, that we are entitled to regard it as, *par excellence*, the Weismannian theory of variation. In the next place, it ought to be observed that Weismann is careful to guard against the seductive fallacy of attributing the origin of sexual propagation to the agency of natural selection. Great as the benefit of this newer mode of propagation must have been to the species presenting it, the benefit cannot have been conferred by natural selection, seeing that the benefit arose from the fact of the new method furnishing material to the operation of natural selection, and therefore constituting the condition to the agency of natural selection having been called into existence at all. Or, in other words, we cannot attribute to natural selection the origin of sexual reproduction without involving ourselves in the absurdity of supposing natural selection to have originated the conditions of its own activity[5]. What the causes may have been which originally led to sexual reproduction is at present a matter that awaits suggestion by way of hypothesis; and, therefore, it now only remains to add that the general structure of Professor Weismann's system of hypotheses leads to this curious result—namely, that the otherwise ubiquitous and (as he supposes) exclusive dominion of natural selection stops short at the protozoa, over which it cannot exercise any influence at all. For if natural selection depends for its activity on the occurrence of congenital variations, and if congenital variations depend for their occurrence on sexual modes of reproduction, it follows that no organisms which propagate by any other modes can present congenital variations, or thus become subject to the sway of natural selection. And inasmuch as Weismann believes that such is the case with all the protozoa, as well as with all parthenogenetic organisms, he does not hesitate to accept the necessary conclusion that in these cases natural selection is without any jurisdiction. How, then, does he account for individual variations in the protozoa? And, still more, how does he account for the origin of their innumerable species? He accounts for both these things by the direct action of external conditions of life. In other words, so far as the unicellular organisms are concerned, Weismann is rigidly and unconditionally an advocate of the theory of Lamarck—just as much as in the case of all the multicellular organisms he is rigidly and unconditionally an opponent of that theory. Nevertheless, there is here no inconsistency: on the contrary, it is consistency with the logical requirements of his theory that leads to this sharp partitioning of the unicellular from the multicellular organisms with respect to the causes of their evolution. For, according to his view, the conditions of propagation among the unicellular organisms are such that parent and offspring are one and the same thing; "the child is a part, and usually a half, of its parent." Therefore, if the parent has been in any way modified by the action of external conditions, it is inevitable that the child should, from the moment of its birth (i.e., fissiparous separation), be similarly modified; and if the modifying influences continue in the same lines for a sufficient length of time, the resulting change of type may become sufficiently pronounced to constitute a new species, genus, &c. But in the case of the multicellular or sexual organisms, the child is not thus merely a severed moiety of its parent; it is the result of the fusion of two highly specialized and extremely minute particles of each of two parents. Therefore, whatever may be thought touching the validity of Weismann's deduction that in no case can any modification induced by external conditions on these parents be transmitted to their progeny, at least we must recognize the validity of the distinction which he draws between the facility with which such transmission must take place in the unicellular organisms, as compared with the difficulty—or, as he believes, the impossibility—of its doing so in the multicellular.

We are now in a position fully to understand Professor Weismann's theory of heredity in all its bearings. Briefly stated, it is as follows. The whole organization of any multicellular organism is composed of two entirely different kinds of cells—namely, the germ-cells, or those which have to do with reproduction, and the somatic-cells, or those which go to constitute all the other parts of the organism. Now, the somatic-cells, in their aggregations as tissues and organs, may be modified in numberless ways by the direct action of the environment, as well as by special habits formed during the individual lifetime of the organism. But although the modifications thus induced may be, and generally are, adaptive—such as the increased muscularity caused by the use of muscles, "practice making perfect" where neural adjustments are concerned, and so on,—in no case can these so-called acquired, or "somatogenetic," characters exercise any influence upon the germ-cells, such that they should reappear in the next generation as congenital, or "blastogenetic," characters. For, according to the theory, the germ-cells as to their germinal contents differ in kind from the somatic-cells, and have no other connexion or dependence upon them than that of deriving from them their food and lodging. So much for the somatic-cells.

Turning now to the germ-cells, these are the receptacles of what Weismann calls the germ-plasm; and this it is that he supposes to differ in kind from all the other constituent elements of the organism. For the germ-plasm he believes to have had its origin in the unicellular organisms, and to have been handed down from them in one continuous stream through all successive generations of multicellular organisms. Thus, for example, suppose that we take a certain *quantum* of germ-plasm as this occurs in any individual organism of to-day. A minute portion of this germ-plasm, when mixed with a similarly minute portion from another individual, goes to form a new individual. But, in doing so, only a portion of this minute portion is consumed; the residue is stored up in the germinal cells of the new individual, in order to secure that continuity of the germ-plasm which Weismann assumes as the necessary basis of his whole theory. Furthermore, he assumes that this overplus portion of germ-plasm, which is so handed over to the custody of the new individual, is there capable of growth or multiplication at the expense of the nutrient materials which are supplied to it by the new soma in which it finds itself located; while in thus growing, or multiplying, it faithfully retains its highly complex structure, so that in no one minute particular does any part of a many thousand-fold increase differ, as to its ancestral characters, from that inconceivably small overplus which was first of all entrusted to the embryo by its parents. Therefore one might represent the germ-plasm by the metaphor of a yeast-plant, a single particle of which may be put into a vat of nutrient fluid: there it lives and grows upon the nutriment supplied, so that a new particle may next be taken to impregnate another vat, and so on *ad infinitum*. Here the successive vats would represent successive generations of progeny; but, to make the metaphor complete, one would have to suppose that in each case the yeast-cell was required to begin by making its own vat of nutrient material, and that it was only the residual portion of the cell which was afterwards able to grow and multiply. But although the metaphor is thus necessarily a clumsy one, it may serve to emphasize the all-important feature of Weismann's theory—namely, the almost absolute independence of the germ-plasm. For, just as the properties of the yeast-plant would be in no way affected by anything that might happen to the vat, short of its being broken up or having its malt impaired, so, according to Weismann, the properties of the germ-plasm cannot be affected by anything that may happen to its containing soma, short of the soma being destroyed or having its nutritive functions disordered.

Such being the relations that are supposed to obtain between the soma and its germ-plasm, we have next to observe what is supposed to happen when, in the course of evolution, some modification of the ancestral form of the soma is required in order to adapt it to some change on the part of its environment. In other words, we have to consider Weismann's views on the *modus operandi* of adaptive development, with its result in the origination of new species.

Seeing that, according to the theory, it is only congenital variations which can be inherited, all variations subsequently acquired by the intercourse of individuals with their environment, however beneficial such variations may be to these individuals, are ruled out as regards the species. Not falling within the province of heredity, they are blocked off in the first generation, and therefore present no significance at all in the process of organic evolution. No matter how many generations of eagles, for instance, may have used their wings for purposes of flight; and no matter how great an increase of muscularity, of endurance, and of skill, may thus have been secured to each generation of eagles as the result of individual exercise; all these advantages are entirely lost to progeny, and young eagles have ever to begin their lives with no more benefit bequeathed by the activity of their ancestors than if those ancestors had all been barn-door fowls. The only material which is of any count as regards the species, or with reference to the process of evolution, are fortuitous variations of the congenital kind. Among all the numberless congenital variations, within narrow limits, which are perpetually occurring in each generation of eagles, some will have reference to the wings; and although these will be fortuitous, or occurring indiscriminately in all directions, a few of them will now and then be in the direction of increased muscularity, others in the direction of increased endurance, others in the direction of increased skill, and so on. Now each of these fortuitous variations, which happens also to be a beneficial variation, will be favoured by natural selection; and, because it likewise happens to be a congenital variation, will be perpetuated by heredity. In the course of time, other congenital variations will happen to arise in the same directions; these will be added by natural selection to the advantage already gained, and so on, till, after hundreds and thousands of generations, the wings of eagles have become evolved into the marvellous structures which they now present.

Such being the theory of natural selection when stripped of all remnants of so-called Lamarckian principles, we have next to consider what the theory means in its relation to germ-plasm. For, as before explained, congenital variations are supposed by Weismann to be due to new combinations taking place in the germ-plasm as a result of the union in every act of fertilisation of two complex hereditary histories. Well, if congenital variations are thus nothing more than variations of germ-plasm "writ large" in the organism which is developed out of the plasm, it follows that natural selection is really at work upon these variations of the plasm. For, although it is proximately at work on the congenital variations of organisms after birth, it is ultimately, and through them, at work upon the variations of germ-plasm out of which the organisms arise. In other words, natural selection, in picking out of each generation those individual organisms which are by their congenital characters best suited to their surrounding conditions of life, is thereby picking out those peculiar combinations or variations of germ-plasm, which, when expanded into a resulting organism, give that organism the best chance in its struggle for existence. And, inasmuch as a certain overplus of this peculiar combination of germ-plasm is entrusted to that organism for bequeathing to the next generation, this to the next, and so on, it follows that natural selection is all the while conserving that originally peculiar combination of germ-plasm, until it happens to meet with some other mass of germ-plasm by mixing with which it may still further improve upon its original peculiarity, when, other things equal, natural selection will seize upon this improvement to perpetuate, as in the previous case. So that, on the whole, we may say that natural selection is ever waiting and watching for such combinations of germ-plasm as will give the resulting organisms the best possible chance in their struggle for existence; while, at the same time, it is remorselessly destroying all those combinations of germ-plasm which are handed over to the custody of organisms not so well fitted to their conditions of life.

It only remains to add that, according to Weismann's theory in its strictly logical form, combinations of germ-plasm when once effected are so stable that they would never alter except as a result of entering into new combinations. In other words, no external influences or internal processes can ever change the hereditary nature of any particular mixture of germ-plasm, save and except its admixture with some other germ-plasm, which, being of a nature equally stable, goes to unite with the first in equal proportions as regards hereditary character. So that really it would be more correct to say that any given mass of germ-plasm does not change even when it is mixed with some other mass—any more, for instance, than a handful of sand can be said to change when it is mixed with a handful of clay.

Consequently, we arrive at this curious result. No matter how many generations of organisms there may have been, and therefore no matter how many combinations of germ-plasm may have taken place to give rise to an existing population, each existing unit of germ-plasm must have remained of the same essential nature or constitution as when it was first started in its immortal career millions of years ago. Or, reverting to our illustration of sand and clay, the particles of each must always remain the same, no matter how many admixtures they may undergo with particles of other materials, such as chalk, slate, &c. Now, inasmuch as it is an essential—because a logically necessary—part of Weismann's theory to assume such absolute stability or unchangeableness on the part of germ-plasm, the question arises, and has to be met, What was the origin of those differences of character in the different germ-plasms of multicellular organisms which first gave rise, and still continue to give rise, to congenital variations by their mixture one with another? This important question Weismann answers by supposing that these differences originally arose out of the differences in the unicellular organisms, which were the ancestors of the primitive multicellular organisms. Now, as before stated, different forms of unicellular organisms are supposed to have originated as so many results of differences in the direct action of the environment. Consequently, according to the theory, all congenital variations which now occur in multicellular organisms, are really the distant results of variations that were aboriginally induced in their unicellular ancestors by the direct action of surrounding conditions of life.

I think it will be well to conclude by briefly summarising the main features of this elaborate theory.

Living material is essentially, or of its own nature, imperishable; and it still continues to be so in the case of unicellular organisms which propagate by fission or gemmation. But as soon as these primitive methods of propagation became, from whatever cause, superseded by sexual, it ceased to be for the benefit of species that their constituent individuals should be immortal; seeing that, if they continued to be so, all species of sexually-reproducing organisms would sooner or later have come to be composed of broken-down and decrepit individuals. Consequently, in all sexually-reproducing or multicellular organisms, natural selection set to work to reduce the term of individual lifetimes within the narrowest limits that in the case of each species were compatible with the procreation and the rearing of progeny. Nevertheless, in all these sexually-reproducing organisms the primitive endowment of immortality has been retained with respect to their germ-plasm, which has thus been continuous, through numberless generations of perishing organisms, from the first origin of sexual reproduction till the present time. Now, it is the union of germ-plasms which is required to reproduce new individuals of multicellular organisms that determines congenital variations on the part of such organisms, and thus furnishes natural selection with the material for its work in the way of organic evolution—work, therefore, which is impossible in the case of unicellular organisms, where variation can never be congenital, but always determined by the direct action of surrounding conditions of life. Again, as the germ-plasm of multicellular organisms is continuous from generation to generation, and at each impregnation gives rise to a more or less novel set of congenital characters, natural selection, in picking out of each generation the congenital characters which are of most service to the organisms presenting them, is really or fundamentally at work upon those variations of the germ-plasm which in turn give origin to these variations of organisms that we recognize as congenital. Therefore, natural selection has always to wait and to watch for such variations of germ-plasm as will eventually prove beneficial to the individuals developed therefrom, who will then transmit this peculiar quality of germ-plasm to their progeny, and so on. Therefore also—and this is most important to remember—natural selection as thus working becomes the one and only cause of organic evolution in all the multicellular organisms, just as the direct action of the environment is the one and only cause of it in the case of all the unicellular organisms. But inasmuch as the multicellular organisms were all in the first instance derived from the unicellular, and inasmuch as their germ-plasm is of so stable a nature that it can never be altered by any agencies internal or external to the organisms presenting it, it follows that all congenital variations are the remote consequences of aboriginal differences on the part of unicellular ancestors. And, lastly, it follows also that these congenital variations— although now so entirely independent of external conditions of life, and even of activities internal to organisms themselves—were originally and exclusively due to the direct action of such conditions on the lives of their unicellular ancestors; while even at the present day no one congenital variation can arise which is not ultimately due to differences impressed upon the protoplasmic substance of the germinal elements, when the parts of which these are now composed constituted integral parts of the protozoa, which were directly and differentially affected by their converse with their several environments.

Again, if for the sake of distinctness we neglect all these far-reaching deductions from his theory of *heredity* whereby Weismann constructs this elaborate theory of *organic evolution*, and fasten our attention only upon the former, we may briefly summarize the fundamental difference between his theory of *heredity* and Darwin's theory of *heredity* thus.

Darwin's theory of heredity is the theory of *Pangenesis*: it supposes that *all* parts of the organism *generate* anew in every individual the formative material which, when collected together in the germ-cells, constitutes the potentiality of a new organism; and that this new organism, when developed, resembles its parents simply because *all* the formative material in each of the parents has been thus *generated* by, and collected from, *all* parts of their respective bodies. Weismann's theory of heredity, on the other hand, is the theory of the *Continuity of Germ-plasm*: it supposes that *no* part of the parent organism generates *any* of the formative material which is to constitute the new organism; but that, on the contrary, this material stands to all the rest of the body in much the same relation as a parasite to its host, showing a life independent of the body, save in so far as the body supplies to it appropriate lodgement and nutrition; that in each generation a small portion of this substance is told off to develop a new body to lodge and nourish the ever-growing and never-dying germ-plasm—this new body, therefore, resembling its so-called parent body simply because it has been developed from one and the same mass of formative material; and, lastly, that this formative material, or germ-plasm, has been continuous through all generations of successively perishing bodies, which therefore stand to it in much the same relation as annual shoots to a perennial stem: the shoots resemble one another simply because they are all grown from one and the same stock.

CHAPTER II.

LATER ADDITIONS TO WEISMANN'S SYSTEM UP TO THE YEAR 1892.

I HAVE now furnished as complete a *résumé* as seems desirable for present purposes of Weismann's theory of germ-plasm, considered both as a theory of heredity and as a sequent theory of organic evolution. But before proceeding to examine this elaborate system as a whole, I must devote another chapter to a further statement of certain later additions to—and also emendations of—the system as it was originally propounded. These additions and alterations have reference only to the theory of heredity: they do not affect the theory of organic evolution as originally deduced therefrom. Moreover they have all been due to our more recently acquired knowledge touching the morphology and physiology of cell-nuclei: it is for the purpose of bringing his theory of germ-plasm into accord with these results of later researches that Weismann has thus modified the theory as it originally stood. For my own part, I do not see that very much is gained by these newer additions and modifications; but, be this as it may, they are certainly very complicated, and on this account I have thought it best to devote a separate chapter to their consideration. Furthermore, not only in the opinion of Weismann himself, but also in that both of his friends and foes, the main question with which his later essays are concerned—viz., as to whether the nucleus of a cell is the only part of a cell which is concerned in the phenomena of heredity—is regarded as of fundamental importance to his entire edifice. Hence, although I cannot myself perceive that the indisputable importance of this question to any speculations on the subject of heredity is of such special or vital significance to Weismann's theory, it becomes necessary for me to supply this further chapter for the purpose of presenting the further developments of his theory.

First of all, Weismann has of late years considerably modified his original view touching the relation of germ-cells to body-cells. For while he originally supposed the fundamental distinction in kind to obtain as between the whole contents of a germ-cell and the whole contents of a somatic-cell, he now regards this distinction as obtaining only between the nucleus of a germ-cell and the nucleus of a somatic-cell. In other words, he regards the whole of a germ-cell, with the exception of its nucleus, as resembling the whole of any other cell, with the exception of *its* nucleus. It is the nucleus of a germ-cell alone that contains germ-plasm: all the rest of such a cell being "nutritive, but not formative."

This transference of the peculiar or hereditary powers of a germ-cell from the cell as a whole to the nucleus, necessitates certain emendations of the original theory of germ-plasm. In particular, the broad distinction between the whole contents of a germ-cell as "germ-plasm," and the whole contents of a somatic-cell as "somato-plasm," is now discarded; and in its stead we have all nuclear matter (whether of germ-cells or somatic-cells) comprised under the one denomination of "nucleo-plasm," in contradistinction to all the other protoplasm of a cell, which is called "cytoplasm." Hence Weismann now regards the cytoplasm of a germ-cell as identical with the cytoplasm of all other cells. Its function is merely that of "nourishing" the nucleus, while, on the other hand, it is "controlled" by the nucleus as to its own growth, shape, size, and eventual division.

But it is evident that the nucleo-plasm of a germ-cell must differ from the nucleo-plasm of a somatic-cell, in that it not only "controls" the growth, &c. of its own cell, but likewise presents all the additional characters peculiar to a germ-cell. That is to say, the nucleo-plasm of a germ-cell resembles the nucleo-plasm of a somatic-cell in that it is nourished by, and exercises control over, the cytoplasm of its own particular cell; but it differs from the nucleo-plasm of a somatic-cell in admitting of fertilization, in the capability of reproducing an entire organism, in the endowing of that organism with all its hereditary characters, and, lastly, in providing for its own reproduction in the next generation.

Thus it is evident, as Weismann puts it, that the nucleo-plasm of a germ-cell must be of *two kinds*—one being concerned with the formation and control of the germ-cell only, while the other has to do with the construction of an entire future organism, and the subsequent reproduction thereof. But not only so; for at each stage in the construction of this future organism, all the somatic-cells, as successively constructed, must likewise contain nucleo-plasm in two kinds—one having to do only with the formation and control of its own individual cell, and the other having to do with the formation of the future somatic-cells, which will have to follow in the course of ontogeny. Therefore, in order to designate this second kind of nucleo-plasm (whether in a germ-cell or a somatic-cell) Weismann borrows from Nägeli the term "idio-plasm[6]," or rather, I should say, he uses the term "nucleo-plasm" when he is speaking of all the contents of a nucleus indiscriminately, while he uses the term "idio-plasm" when he has occasion to speak specially of the two kinds of nucleo-plasm now before us.

Hence, the nuclear contents (nucleo-plasm) of every cell, whether germinal or somatic, present two substances, which we may, in the absence of any better terms supplied by Weismann himself, respectively designate "idio-plasm-A" and "idio-plasm-B." Idio-plasm-A is the substance which has to do only with the formation and control of the individual cell in which it resides, like a mollusc in its shell. Idio-plasm-B is the substance out of which future cells are to be formed and controlled, when in due course either of ontogeny or phylogeny this idio-plasm-B becomes converted into idio-plasm-A,—i.e., into each subsequently developing tissue or organism, as the case may be. I say ontogeny or phylogeny, and tissue or organism, because, where a *germ-cell* is concerned, idio-plasm-B is capable of reproducing entire organisms of its own and of subsequent generations; whereas, in the case of all *somatic*-cells, idio-plasm-B is capable only of reproducing, stage by stage, some greater or less number of the cells which are to construct the single organism of which they form a part. Or, otherwise expressed, in the particular case of a germ-cell idio-plasm-B is germ-plasm, and therefore is alone capable of producing an entire organism of somatic-cells, while it is likewise alone capable of reproducing successive organisms; for it alone contains the carriers of heredity[7].

Thus, idio-plasm-B of an unsegmented germ-nucleus is germ-plasm. But as soon as the germ-nucleus has undergone its first nuclear division, its nucleo-plasm is no longer germ-plasm, inasmuch as each of the half-portions is now no longer capable of reproducing an entire organism—unless it be in the case of identical twins. Similarly in the second nuclear division, each of the four resulting idio-plasms-B is still further removed from the pristine character of germ-plasm; and so on through all successive stages of segmentation. Hence these successive nuclear divisions must indicate a partitioning and re-partitioning of the original idio-plasm-B (germ-plasm) into the idio-plasms-B severally distinctive of all the various cells of the soma.

Now, it is evident that not *all* the idio-plasm-B of a germ-cell which thus passes over into the nuclei of somatic-cells can be represented by the idio-plasm-B of those cells. At every stage of successive cell-formation a certain part of the original idio-plasm-B of the germ-cell must become the idio-plasm-A of somatic-cells distinctive of that stage. For, supposing that at its differentiation stage 99 the original germ-plasm (now somatic-idio-plasm-B of 99th stage) has reached a phase of ontogeny where the formation of tissue *m* has next to be followed by the formation of tissue *n*, then there still remain the further differentiation stages 101, 102, 103, &c., to be provided for, which, when their time arrives, will go to form the still later tissues *o, p, q,* &c. Consequently the idio-plasm-B of stage 100 cannot be *all* consumed in making the tissue *n*. There must be a residual portion which will afterwards be called upon to form successively the idio-plasm-A of *o, p, q,* &c. Where, then, is this residual portion of idio-plasm posited? Clearly it must be posited in the nuclei of *n*. Thus it is that, as we began by stating, all the nuclei of any given tissue *n* really contain two kinds of substance,—(1) their own idio-plasm-A, which was part of idio-plasm-B of the preceding tissue, *m*; and (2) the idio-plasm-B, which is destined to become idio-plasms-A of succeeding tissues *o, p, q,* &c. Thus it follows also that the more the original idio-plasm-B is differentiated into these successive formations of idio-plasms-A the less of it remains for further differentiation, till, at the last stage of ontogeny, all the original idio-plasm-B (germ-plasm) has been thus changed into idio-plasms-A severally distinctive of all the somatic-tissues *a*, *b*, *c*—*x*, *y*, *z*,—save only the portion of it which has been carried through all these ontogenetic stages in a wholly *un*differentiated condition, for the purpose of securing the *phylogenetic* production of the next generation. And this, of course, is secured by the portion of undifferentiated germ-plasm in question being deposited in the nuclei of germ-cells, at whatever stage of the ontogeny these may be formed.

Finally, it is evident that, *at each stage* of the differentiation of idio-plasm-B into idio-plasms-A, the portion concerned must be capable of self-multiplication to an almost incalculable extent,—yet this only as idio-plasm-B of the particular kind required for constructing the idio-plasm-A which is appropriate to the particular stage. Such is a necessary deduction from the terms of Weismann's theory, inasmuch as we know that at each of the ontogenetic stages there is an incalculable multiplication of cells belonging to that stage—cells, the "cytoplasm" of which necessarily presupposes for its formation its own appropriate idio-plasm in both kinds, and this in similarly increased quantities.

From the above theory it follows that an explanation can be given of the healing of wounds (as in ourselves), of the regeneration of lost parts (as the limb of a newt), or even of the reproduction of an entire organism from a mere fragment of somatic-tissue (as in the cases already alluded to at the commencement of this chapter—viz. the leaf of Begonia, portions of sea-anemones, jelly-fish, &c.). For in all these cases of repair, regeneration, and what may be called *somatic reproduction*, we have only to suppose that not all the idio-plasm-B of any given ontogenetic stage is consumed in the formation of that stage, and therefore that the residue is passed on to the later stages *in a latent condition*. It will then be available at any time to re-develop tissue corresponding to that particular stage, should that particular tissue happen to be lost by accident or disease. For example, if some of the idio-plasm-B of the very first ontogenetic stage, or true germ-plasm, should thus be passed on in an undifferentiated condition through the somatic-tissues subsequently formed at later ontogenetic stages, then we can understand why an *entire* organism is reproduced from a fragment of these tissues—or of those among which particles of such residual and undifferentiated germ-plasm happen to be scattered. Similarly, if idio-plasm-B of the ontogenetic stage at which a limb is formed be not all consumed in constructing the limb, then the limb, if afterwards lost, will be reconstructed, although an entire organism will not be reproduced from a fragment of somatic-tissue. And similarly also with the mere repair of injuries, where the only overplus of idio-plasm-B is that of idio-plasm-B belonging to the very last stages of ontogeny.

But, it is almost needless to observe, this kind of transmission of idio-plasm-B from one stage of ontogeny in an unaltered condition to subsequent stages, is not to be confused with the other kind of transmission previously referred to, whereby idio-plasm-B of one stage becomes successively transformed into the idio-plasms-A of successive stages. In the former case, at whatever stage of ontogeny the transmission may start from, the idio-plasm-B from that stage lies dormant, and is never destined to undergo further differentiation, unless the results of accident or disease should call upon it to do so. In the latter case, on the other hand, the idio-plasm-B of any given stage is passed on to the next stage for the express purpose of transforming itself into the idio-plasms-A of that and, in due order, of all subsequent stages.

It will be observed that all this elaboration of the original theory of germ-plasm—an elaboration which is largely derived from the speculative writings of Nägeli—serves no other purpose than that of indicating what Professor Weismann now regards as the most probable *mode* in which germ-plasm undergoes its modification into the various kinds of somatic-cells. For, inasmuch as the idio-plasms-B of all somatic-cells are originally derived from that of the germ-cell, and inasmuch as each expends its formative energies exclusively in constructing and controlling the cells which, as idio-plasms-A, they respectively inhabit, it is still the germ-plasm of the original germ-cell that is finally converted into the various tissues which together constitute the soma—notwithstanding that, in order thus to become transmuted into body-substance, or somato-plasm,it must pass through the sundry intermediate stages of idio-plasm-B, idio-plasm-A, and cytoplasm, of any given ontogenetic stage. Hence I do not see that it makes any substantial difference to Weismann's theory of heredity, whether we speak of germ-plasm being converted into "somato-plasm," or into "idio-plasm" *plus* "somatic-idio-plasm," *plus* "cytoplasm." But as Weismann himself thinks that it does make some great difference whether we adhere to his original generic term "somato-plasm," or adopt his newer and more specific terms as just enumerated, I append *in extenso* the most recent exposition of his views upon this subject[8].

Before quitting this somewhat complicated addition to the original theory of germ-plasm, I must briefly allude to the descriptions and illustrations of karyokinesis which were given in Part I of *Darwin and after Darwin*, for the prospective benefit of any general readers who might afterwards be sufficiently interested in Weismann's speculations to desire a statement of the main facts on which this further development of his theory rests. It seemed undesirable to burden the present volume with an account of recent investigations so well known to naturalists, while, on the other hand, it was clearly desirable that such an account should be given somewhere, if the speculations in question were to be rendered intelligible to anybody else. Therefore I must here request those of my readers who are not already acquainted with the matter to consult pp. 128-134 of Part I. It will there be seen how enormously complex are the visible processes which take place in the nucleus of a germ-cell (and likewise of a somatic-cell), preparatory to its division; and therefore, supposing that the nucleus alone contains the material concerned in the phenomena of heredity, it appears that no small corroboration is lent to Weismann's views by these histological observations. And, more particularly, if we suppose with him that the material in question is restricted to that portion of the segregating nuclear matter which is called the "nuclear thread[9]," in the formation of the "loops" or "rods" of this substance we seem to have presented a visible expression of the marshalling of "the carriers of heredity," and the successive passage of the originally generalized "germ-plasm" of the germ-cell into the ever more and more specialized "nucleo-plasms" of the somatic-cells. Indeed, the new theory of heredity, when thus brought into relation with the new results of histological observation, appears so well to fit the latter, that one would be sorry to find the coincidence unmeaning, or the theory false. But, without passing any criticism, it is sufficient to note that the question whether or not the theory is true—and therefore correctly interprets the phenomena of karyokinesis,—must depend chiefly on whether it be eventually proved that the "nuclear thread" is indeed the only part of a germ-cell, or even the only part of a tissue-cell, which is concerned in controlling the phenomena of heredity on the one hand, and of ontogeny on the other. Into this question, however, I do not propose to enter. It will be enough to assume, for the sake of argument, that Weismann's view of the matter will eventually prove to be true. At the same time, we must remember that at present this view as to the nuclear thread being the sole repository of the material of heredity is merely hypothetical.

We now arrive at the last of those features in Weismann's theory of heredity, the importance of which necessitates mention in such a mere statement of the theory as the present chapter is concerned with.

According to Weismann's own view of his theory, two objections have to be met. In the first place, there is the objection that all individuals *which are born of the same parents* are not exactly alike, as the theory might have expected they would be, seeing that the admixture of identical germ-plasms has been concerned in the formation of the whole progeny. In the second place, and quite apart from this objection, there is the difficulty that, if every act of fertilization essentially consists in a fusion of one mass of germ-plasm belonging to a male germ-cell with another mass belonging to a female germ-cell, at each generation the mass of germ-plasm contained in an egg-cell must be doubled—with the result that ova must progressively increase in size during the course of phylogeny. But ova do not thus progressively increase in size. Therefore, if the imperishable nature of germ-plasm is to be theoretically sustained, it is necessary to show some means whereby ova and spermatozoa are able to get rid of at least one half of their respective germ-plasms in each generation—i.e., before each act of impregnation. Weismann meets both these difficulties by an appeal to the following facts.

It is well known that the ripe ovum extrudes two minute particles of protoplasmic substance, which are called polar bodies[10]. These both proceed from the nucleus of the ovum, but are not formed simultaneously. For the first polar body is really one half of the original nucleus of the cell, and therefore is formed by the first segmentation of this nucleus. The second polar body, on the other hand, is one half of the remaining nucleus, and is similarly formed by the second segmentation. Hence, when both polar bodies have been extruded from the ovum, only one quarter of the original nuclear matter remains. So far, of course, the facts prove too much for Weismann's theory, because the theory wants to get rid of only one half of the original nuclear matter before impregnation, *if all the nuclear matter be germ-plasm*. Therefore Weismann concludes that all the original nuclear matter of the ripe ovum is not germ-plasm, but that only one half of it is so, while the other half—or that half which goes to constitute the first polar body—is idio-plasm-A, which, as we have already seen, the egg-cell shares in common with all other cells. It is merely "ovogenetic": its function is that of constructing the ovum, *quâ* cell: it has nothing whatever to do with the germ-plasm which the particular cell contains. Therefore, having discharged its function of constructing this cell, it is itself discharged from the cell as the first polar body.

The nucleus of the fully-formed ovum having thus got rid of all its superfluous idio-plasm-A by throwing off the first polar body, is supposed henceforth to consist of pure germ-plasm (i.e., of idio-plasm-B belonging to the first ontogenetic stage), and one half of this is next got rid of by the second segmentation in the form of the second polar body. Therefore, according to the theory and so far as the problems of heredity are concerned, we need not any further trouble ourselves about the first polar body. But it will at once be seen that by the interpretation which Weismann puts upon the second polar body, and also, of course, upon the extrusion of some of its nuclear matter by the male cell, he meets both the difficulties against his theory of germ-plasm which we are now engaged in considering.

That he thus meets the second of those difficulties—i.e., concerning the otherwise perpetual accumulation of germ-plasm—is evident without explanation. That he likewise meets the first—i.e., concerning the non-resemblance of individuals born of the same parents—is scarcely less evident. For it is hardly conceivable that such a complex mass of germ-plasms as the nucleus of a fertilized ovum must be could ever present in any two eggs precisely the same proportional representation of the "carriers of heredity," after one half of each set had been thus discharged from each egg. Therefore, if the second polar body removes from each egg one half of the ancestral germ-plasms, "every egg will contain a somewhat different combination of hereditary tendencies, and thus the offspring which arise from the different germ-cells of the same mother can never be identical[11].

Such, then, is Weismann's theory of the physiological meaning of polar bodies. And as the bearing of this particular theory on his more general theory of heredity does not appear to me a vitally intimate one, I think my subsequent examination of the main theory will be simplified if I now proceed at once to an examination of the subordinate one. For by doing this I shall hope to show that the bearings just mentioned are of much less importance than he represents them to be; and, therefore, that we may hereafter proceed to consider his theory of heredity without any special reference to his theory of polar bodies.

To begin with, as regards the first polar body, one would like to know more clearly why it is necessary that this residuum of merely "ovogenetic idio-plasm" (or idio-plasm-A of the egg-cell) has to be got rid of before the germ-plasm can proceed to discharge its physiological functions. Seeing that both these (hypothetically) very different materials occur in the self-same nucleus, some very delicate mechanism must be needed for their separation; and it is not apparent why such a mechanism should have been evolved, rather than what would have been the simpler plan of adapting the germ-plasm to hold its own against the idio-plasm-A, even if one could see that any interference between these very different substances is in any way probable. For my own part, at all events, I cannot see why this microscopical atom of "ovogenetic idio-plasm" should not simply be left to be absorbed among the millions of cells that afterwards go to form the foetus.

Again, as regards the second polar body, Weismann's theory of it is framed to explain, (a) how the excess of germ-plasm is got rid of in each ontogeny, and (b) why the offspring of the same parents do not all precisely resemble one another. These, be it observed, are the only two functions which Weismann's theory of polar bodies subserves in relation to his theory of germ-plasm. But, it appears to me, neither of these functions is necessary, in so far as any requirements of the latter theory are concerned. For surely, polar bodies or no polar bodies, there is already a mechanism at work in each ontogeny which is of itself sufficient to discharge both these functions, and so to anticipate both the supposed difficulties which the subsidiary theory is adduced to meet. The very essence of ontogeny, as a process, itself consists in a continuous succession of nuclear divisions—and this not only as regards somatic-cells, but also as regards germ-cells. Now, in the great majority of organisms, there is an infinitely greater number of germ-cells (both male and female) than can possibly be required either for the purpose of getting rid of any excess of germ-plasms in the nucleus of each cell, or of preventing the

25

germ-plasms of any one germ-cell precisely resembling those of any other. If every plant or animal produced only a single female-cell or a single male-cell, then indeed we might require from Professor Weismann a demonstration of some special mechanism to secure the expulsion of half its ancestral germ-plasms; since otherwise the single female-cell or male-cell would have to increase its dimensions in each successive generation. But, as matters actually stand, nature seems to have made much more than ample provision for preventing the undue accumulation of ancestral germ-plasms in any individual germ-cell, by enormously multiplying; through continuous division and subdivision, the *number* of germ-cells in each ontogeny. And similarly, of course, as regards the different aggregations of ancestral germ-plasms which are left for distribution among these innumerable germ-cells. "If one group of ancestral germ-plasms is expelled from one egg, and a different group from another egg, it follows that no two eggs can be exactly alike as regards their contained hereditary tendencies." Granted; but this consideration applies equally to the original segregation of germ-plasms in the multiplying eggs of each ontogeny—for it follows from the theory of germ-plasm that the most primitive egg-cell in each ontogeny must have contained all the ancestral germ-plasms which are afterwards distributed among its innumerable progeny of egg-cells. And, as far as the facts of "individual variation" are concerned, I do not see why the differential partitioning of "ancestral idio-plasms" should be any better secured by nuclear division of a mature germ-cell than by that of an immature. Less so, indeed; for the wonder is that during the many-thousand-fold division of an immature ovum so precise a distribution of these "ancestral idio-plasms" is maintained, as is proved to be maintained (on the theory of germ-plasm) by the facts of heredity.

However, Weismann takes a widely different view of the matter. For while he allows that "such an early reducing division would offer advantages in that nothing would be lost, for both the daughter nuclei would (? might) become eggs, instead of one of them being lost as a polar body"—while he allows this, he nevertheless rejects the possibility of "such an early reducing division." But I do not see that the reasons which he assigns for this rejection of it are adequate.

First, he says that if this were the way in which the superfluous germ-plasm of each generation were got rid of, *far too much* provision has been made for the purpose,— seeing that the practically indefinite number of nuclear divisions which the immature germ-cells undergo would cause a much "greater decrease of the ancestral idio-plasms of each than could afterwards be compensated by the increase due to fertilization." But this rejoinder is of cogency only if it be supposed that at each nuclear division of an immature ovum, "the ancestral idio-plasms" (germ-plasm) are incapable of the power of self-multiplication which soon afterwards becomes one of its most essential characters. Why, then, should we suppose this substance to be totally incapable of increase in the multiplying ova of ontogeny, when at the same time we are to suppose the same substance capable of any amount of increase in the multiplying ova of phylogeny? To this obvious question no answer is supplied: in fact the question is not put.

Secondly, Weismann says that in parthenogenetic ova only one polar body is extruded. This he regards as equivalent to the first polar body of a fertilizable ovum (i.e., as composed of ovogenetic nuclear substance); and hence he argues that the second polar body of a fertilizable ovum must be regarded as composed of germ-plasm. But even supposing that he is right as to the fact that parthenogenetic ova invariably extrude but one polar body, his argument from this fact would only be available after we had already accepted his view touching the character of the second polar body. So long as this view is itself the subject of debate, he cannot prove it by the fact in question. In other words, unless we have already agreed that the second polar body has the function which Weismann assigns to it, we cannot accept the fact which he adduces as furnishing any evidence of his view touching the function of the second polar body.

For these reasons I cannot see that the subordinate theory of polar bodies is required in the interests of the general theory of germ-plasm. The difficulties which it is adduced to meet do not appear to me to be any difficulties at all. Therefore, in now proceeding to consider what in my opinion are the real difficulties which lie against the major theory of germ-plasm, I shall not again allude to the minor—and, in this connexion, superfluous—theory of polar bodies.

Such, then, is Professor Weismann's theory of heredity in its original and strictly logical form. In the course of our examination of it which is to follow in Chapter III and IV, we shall find that in almost every one of its essential features, as above stated, the theory has had to undergo—or is demonstrably destined to undergo—some radical modification. But I have thought it best to begin by presenting the whole theory in its completely connected state, as it is in this way alone that we shall be able to disconnect what I regard as the untenable parts from the parts which still remain for investigation at the hands of biological science. Such, indeed, is the only object of my "Examination of Weismannism." For, rightly or wrongly, it appears to me that the unquestionable value of his elaborate speculations is seriously discounted by certain oversights with regard to matters of fact, and not a few inconsistencies touching matters of theory. In displaying both these defects, I am not without hope that the result may be that of inducing Professor Weismann so to modify his system of theories as to strengthen the whole by removing its weaker parts.

CHAPTER III.

WEISMANN'S THEORY OF HEREDITY (1891).

WE now proceed to examine Weismann's theory of germ-plasm, and as this in its various developments has now become a highly complex theory, we had best begin by marking out the lines on which the examination will be conducted.

As I have already pointed out, the Weismannian system is not concerned only with the physiology of reproduction: it is concerned also—and in an even larger measure—with the doctrine of descent. The theory of germ-plasm as a whole is very much more than a theory of heredity; it is a new theory of evolution. The latter, indeed, is deduced from the former; but although the two are thus intimately related, they are nevertheless not mutually dependent. For the relationship is such that the new theory of evolution stands upon the basis supplied by the new theory of heredity, and although it follows from this that if the latter were disproved the former would collapse, it does not follow that if the former were to be found untenable the latter must necessarily be negatived. Hence, for the sake of clearness, and also for the sake of doing justice to both theories, we had best deal with them separately. The present chapter, then, will be devoted to examining Weismann's theory of heredity, while the ensuing chapter will be concerned with his sequent theory of evolution.

Again, Weismann's theory of heredity stands on his fundamental postulate—the continuity of germ-plasm; and also on a fact well recognized by all other theories of heredity, which he calls the stability of germ-plasm. But his sequent theory of evolution stands not only on this fundamental postulate, and on this well-recognized fact; it requires for its logical basis two further postulates—viz., that germ-plasm has been *perpetually* continuous "since the first origin of life," and *unalterably* stable "since the first origin of sexual propagation." That these things are so, a very few words will be sufficient to prove.

Any theory of heredity which supposes the material of heredity to occupy a more or less separate "sphere" of its own, is not obliged further to suppose that this material has *always* been thus isolated, or even that it is now *invariably* so. There have been one or two such theories prior to Weismann's, and they were founded on the well-known fact of congenital characters being at any rate *much more* heritable than are acquired characters. But it has not been needful for these theories to assume that the "continuity" thus postulated has been *perpetually* unbroken. Even if it has been frequently to some extent interrupted, all the facts of *heredity* could be equally well comprised under such theories—and this even if it be supposed that acquired characters are but rarely, or never, transmitted to progeny. For, in as far as the continuity may have been interrupted, it does not follow that the acquired characters (body-changes), which by hypothesis caused the interruption, must be inherited by progeny exactly as they occurred in the parents. Or, in other words and adopting Weismann's terminology, *so far as the facts of heredity are concerned*, there is no reason why germ-plasm should not frequently have had its hereditary qualities modified by some greater or less degree of commerce with somatic-tissues, and yet never have reproduced in progeny the identical acquired characters which caused the modification of germ-plasm in the parents: some other and totally different characters might with equal—or even more—likelihood have been the result, as we shall see more clearly a few pages further on. Why, then, does Weismann so insist upon this continuity of germ-plasm as *perpetual* "since the origin of life"? It appears to me that his only reason for doing so is to provide a basis, not for his theory of heredity, but for his additional theory of evolution. It is of no consequence to the former that germ-plasm should be regarded as thus perpetual, while it is of high importance to the latter that the fundamental postulate of continuity should be supplemented by this further postulate of the continuity as thus perpetual.

Similarly as regards the postulate of the stability of germ-plasm as absolute. It is enough for all the requirements of Weismann's theory of heredity that the material basis of heredity should present a merely *high degree* of stability, such as the facts of atavism, degeneration, &c. abundantly prove that it possesses. For his sequent theory of evolution, however, it is necessary to postulate this stability as *absolute* "since the first origin of sexual reproduction." Otherwise there would be no foundation for any of the distinctive doctrines which go to constitute this theory.

It may not be immediately apparent that Weismann's theory of heredity is not *per se* concerned with either of these two additional postulates of the continuity of germ-plasm as *perpetual*, and the stability of germ-plasm as *absolute*; while both are logically necessary to his further theory of evolution. On this account, and also for the sake of clearness in all that is to follow, we had best begin by comparing his theory of heredity with those of his principal predecessors—Darwin and Galton.

For the purposes of this comparison we may start by again alluding to the fact, that even in the multicellular organisms reproduction is not confined to the sexual methods. Many kinds of invertebrated animals will reproduce entire organisms from the fragments into which a single organism has been chopped: plants of various kinds can be propagated indefinitely by cuttings, grafts, and buds, or even by leaves, as we have already observed in Chapter I. Now, when the whole organism is thus reproduced from a severed portion of somatic-tissue, it reproduces its sexual elements. Whence, then, in such cases are these elements derived? Obviously they are not derived immediately from the sexual organs—or even from the sexual cells—of their parents: they are derived from the somatic-cells of a single parent, if we choose to retain this term; and therefore, as Strasburger pointed out soon after Weismann's theory was published, it seems as if such facts are in themselves destructive of the theory. How, then, does Weismann meet them? As we have already seen in Chapter II, he meets them in the only way they can be met on the lines of his theory—viz., by those newer amendments of his theory which suppose that in all these cases the germ-plasm is *not* confined to the specially sexual cells, but occurs also in the nuclear substance of those somatic-cells which thus prove themselves capable of developing into entire organisms. In other words, the sexual elements which develop during what I have previously called this "somatic reproduction" of multicellular organism, are supposed to be derived from the sexual cells of ancestors, not indeed immediately (for this they plainly are not), but mediately through the somatic-tissues of their a-sexual parent. Now, in view of this extension, the theory of germ-plasm becomes somewhat closely allied to that of pangenesis. For example, when the fragment of a leaf of *Begonia* is laid upon moist soil, there strikes root, and grows a new *Begonia* plant capable of sexual reproduction, Darwin supposes the explanation to be that what he calls "formative material" occurs in all cells of the leaf, while Weismann supposes the explanation to be that what he calls "germ-plasm " occurs in all—or at any rate in most—of the cells of the leaf. So that, except as regards the terms employed, the two theories are identical in their mode of viewing this particular class of phenomena.

Moreover by thus allowing, in his second essay on Heredity, that germ-plasm need not be restricted to the specially sexual cells, but in some cases, at any rate[12], may occur distributed in full measure of reproductive efficiency throughout the general tissues of the organism, Weismann cannot refrain from taking the further step of supposing that the germ-plasm, like the gemmules of Darwin, is capable of any amount of multiplication *in the general cellular tissues of plants*—seeing that plants can be propagated by cuttings, buds, &c., indefinitely. And this, as we have seen, Professor Weismann, in his second essay, does not shrink from doing. Moreover, although I cannot remember that he has anywhere expressly said so, it is obvious that the allied phenomena of regeneration and repair admit of explanation by his hypothesis of "ontogenetic grades," after the manner already stated in Chapter II. Indeed, it is evident that in no other way can these phenomena be brought within the range of his theory. But from this it follows that not only in the case of organisms which are capable of somatic reproduction is the formative nucleo-plasm (idio-plasm-B) diffused throughout the somatic-tissues: on the contrary, it must be *universally* diffused throughout *all* the somatic-cells of *all* living organisms; and whether as it there occurs it is capable of reproducing entire organisms, single organs, single tissues, or a mere cicatrix, depends only on the "ontogenetic grade" of differentiation which this diffused nucleo-plasm has (or has not) previously undergone. Moreover, as we have already seen, at whatever ontogenetic grade of differentiation it may be present in a given somatic-tissue, it must there be capable of indefinite self-multiplication. Therefore, in all these respects this "formative nucleo-plasm" (or idio-plasm-B) of Weismann precisely resembles the "formative material" (or gemmules) of Darwin.

Lastly, as De Vries has pointed out[13], there must be at least as many divisions and subdivisions in the substance of germ-plasm, as there are differences between the somatic organs, tissues, and even cells, to which germ-plasm eventually gives rise—no matter through how many ontogenetic grades of idio-plasm it may first have to pass. Or, in other words, we must accept, as the material basis of heredity, ultimate particles[14] of germ-plasm, which are already differentiated into as many diverse categories as there are differences between all the constituent parts of the resulting soma; for, as shown in the Appendix, no change in the facts of the case has been shown by simply changing the original term "germ-plasm" into "idio-plasm," wherever the phenomena of ontogeny are concerned. It may be convenient, for the sake of presenting newer additions to the theory, to restrict the term "germ-plasm" to "idio-plasm of the first ontogenetic stage"; but as idio-plasms of all subsequent ontogenetic stages are supposed to be ultimately derived from this idio-plasm of the first stage, it is evident that the particulate differences in question must already have been present in the so-called "undifferentiated idio-plasm of the first ontogenetic stage." Unless we are to have a mere juggling with words, we cannot put into our successive idio-plasms any particles of kinds differing from those which are contained in the original germ-plasm. Therefore I say that, notwithstanding this change of terminology, Weismann must continue to assume, as the material basis of heredity, ultimate particles of germ-plasm which are already differentiated into as many diverse categories as there are differences between the parts of the resulting soma—although, of course, these ultimate particles need not be nearly so numerous *in each of their categories* as they afterwards become by self-multiplication while forming each of the resulting tissues.

But this is precisely what the theory of pangenesis supposes; so that I see no reason why these ultimate particles of germ-plasm should not be regarded as "gemmules," so far as their *size, number,* and *function* are concerned. In point of fact, they differ from gemmules only in respect to their *origin*: they are not particles derived from somatic-cells of the preceding generation, but particles derived from germ-plasm of the preceding generation. Or, to state the difference in another form, if we regard the sexual elements as constituting the physiological centre of the organism, then the theory of germ-plasm supposes these ultimate carriers of heredity to originate at this centre, and then to travel centrifugally; while the theory of pangenesis supposes them to originate at the periphery, and then to travel centripetally.

This point of difference, however, arises from the deeper ones, which—having now exhausted the points of agreement—we must next proceed to state.

If, as we have seen, "formative material" and "germ-plasm" agree in being particulate; in constituting the material basis of heredity; in being mainly lodged in highly specialized, or germinal, cells; in being nevertheless also distributed throughout the general cellular tissues, where they are alike concerned in all processes of regeneration, repair, and a-sexual reproduction; in having an enormously complex structure, so that every constituent part of the future organism is already represented in them by corresponding particles; in being everywhere capable of a virtually unlimited multiplication, without ever losing their hereditary endowments; in often carrying these endowments in a dormant state through a number of generations, until at last they reappear again in what we recognize as reversions to ancestral characters;—if in all these most important respects the two substances are supposed to be alike, it may well appear at first sight that there is not much room left for any difference between them. And, in point of fact, the only difference that does obtain between them admits of being stated in two words,—Continuity, and Stability. Nevertheless, although thus so few in number, these two points of difference are points of great importance, as I will now proceed briefly to show.

If the substance which constitutes the material basis of heredity has been *perpetually continuous*, in the sense of never having had any of its hereditary endowments in any way affected by the general body-tissues in which it resides, the following important consequences, it will be remembered, arise. The process of organic evolution must have been exclusively due to a natural selection of favourable variations occurring within the limits of this substance itself; and therefore the so-called Lamarckian factors can never have played any part at all in the evolution of any but the unicellular organisms. On the other hand, if this substance has not been thus perpetually continuous, but more or less formed anew at each ontogeny by the general body-tissues in which it resides, natural selection has probably been in some corresponding degree assisted in its work of organic evolution by the Lamarckian factors, with the result that the experiences of parents count for something in the congenital endowments of their offspring. So much for the first of the two differences between germ-plasm and gemmules, or the difference which arises from the perpetual continuity of germ-plasm.

Touching the second difference, or that which arises from the *absolute stability* of germ-plasm, it will be remembered how from this character there arises another important chain of consequences. Namely, individual variations of the congenital kind can only be due to admixtures of different masses of germ-plasm in every act of sexual fertilization; natural selection is therefore dependent, for the possibility of its working, upon the sexual methods of propagation; hence, natural selection is without any jurisdiction among the unicellular organisms, where the Lamarckian factors hold exclusive sway; and hence, also, the multicellular organisms are ultimately dependent upon this absolute stability of their germ-plasm for all the progress which they have made in the past, as well as for any progress which they may be destined to make in the future.

Thus we see that the two points of difference between germ-plasm and gemmules are not merely of great importance as regards the particular problem which is presented by the phenomena of heredity: they are of still greater importance as regards the general theory of evolution. For if these two qualities of perpetual continuity and absolute stability can be proved to belong to the material basis of heredity, the entire theory of evolution will have to be reconstructed from its very foundation—and this quite apart from the more special question as to the transmission of acquired characters. Therefore we shall presently have to consider these two alleged qualities with the care that they demand, as having been seriously suggested by so eminent a naturalist as Professor Weismann. But, before proceeding to do so, I must briefly compare his theory with that of Mr. Galton.

31

"Stirp" resembles both "germ-plasm" and "gemmules" in all the respects which have above been named as common to the two latter. But it differs from gemmules and further resembles germ-plasm in all the following particulars. It is derived from the stirp of proceeding generations, and constitutes the sole basis of heredity. Only a part of it, however, is consumed in each ontogeny—the residue being handed over to "contribute to form the stirps of the offspring," where it undergoes self-multiplication at the expense of the nutriment supplied to it from the somatic system of the offspring, and so on through successive generations. Again, stirp is concerned in all processes of regeneration and repair, in the same centrifugal manner as germ-plasm is so concerned. Furthermore, the influence of sexual propagation in the blending of hereditary qualities of the stirp is recognized, while the principle of panmixia, or the cessation of selection, is entertained, and shown to invalidate the evidence of pangenesis which Darwin derived from the apparently transmitted effects of use and disuse in our domesticated animals[15]. Lastly, it is clearly stated that on the basis supplied by this "theory of heredity," it becomes logically possible to dispense with the Lamarckian principles *in toto*, leaving natural selection as the sole known cause of organic evolution through a perpetual continuity of stirp, together with individual variations of the same, whether by sexual admixture or otherwise.

So far, then, there is not merely resemblance, but virtual identity, between the theories of stirp and germ-plasm. Disregarding certain speculative details, the coincidence is as complete as that between a die and its impress. But although the two theories are thus similar in *logical construction*, they differ in their interpretations of *biological fact*. That is to say, although Galton anticipated by some ten years all the main features of Weismann's theory of heredity[16], and showed that, as a matter of form, it was logically intact, he refrained from concluding on this account that it must be the true theory of heredity. He argued, indeed, that in the main it was probably the true theory; but he guarded his presentation of it by not undertaking to deny that there might still be some degree of intercommunication between the material basis of heredity in stirp, and the somatic tissues of successive organisms. The construction of a theory which, as a matter of theory, could dispense with the Lamarckian principles *in toto*, was seen to be a very different thing from proving, as a matter of fact, that these principles are non-existent—and this, even though it was seen that a recognition of the principle of panmixia must be taken to have considerably attenuated the *degree* of their operation as previously estimated by Darwin in the theory of pangenesis. In short, after pointing out that the doctrine of stirp might very well adopt the position which about a decade later was adopted by the doctrine of germ-plasm—namely, that of altogether *supplanting* the doctrine of gemmules,—Galton allowed that this could be done only as a matter of formal speculation; and that, as a matter of real interpretation of the facts of nature, it seemed more judicious to stop at *modifying* the doctrine of gemmules, by provisionally retaining the hypothesis of gemmules, but assigning to their agency a greatly subordinate *rôle*. Or to quote his own words:—

> The conclusion to be drawn from the foregoing arguments is, that we might almost reserve our belief that the structural [i. e., "somatic"] cells can react on the sexual elements at all, and we may be confident that at the most they do so in a very faint degree; in other words, that acquired modifications are barely, if at all, inherited, in the correct sense of that word. If they were not heritable, then the second group of cases [i.e., those of acquired as distinguished from congenital

32

characters] would vanish, and we should be absolved from all further trouble; if they exist, in however faint a degree, a complete theory of heredity must account for them. I propose, as already stated, to accept the supposition of their being faintly heritable, and to account for them by a modification of Pangenesis[17].

Seeing, then, that Galton did not undertake to deny a possibly slight influence of somatic-tissues on the hereditary qualities of stirp, it follows that he did not have to proceed to those drastic modifications of the general theory of descent which Weismann has attempted. Stirp, like germ-plasm, is *continuous*; but, unlike germ-plasm, it is not *necessarily* or *absolutely* so. Again, stirp, like germ-plasm, is *stable*; yet, unlike germ-plasm, it is not *perpetually* or *unalterably* so. Hence we hear nothing from Galton about our having to explain the unlikeness of our children to ourselves by variations in our protozoan ancestors; nor do we meet with any of those other immense reaches of deductive speculation which, in my opinion, merely disfigure the republication of stirp under the name of germ-plasm.

Now, I allude to these, the only important points of difference between stirp and germ-plasm, for the sake of drawing prominent attention to the fact that it makes a literally immeasurable difference whether we suppose the material basis of heredity to be *perpetually* continuous and *unalterably* stable, or whether we suppose that it is but *largely* continuous and *highly* stable. In the former case, all the far-reaching deductions which Weismann draws with reference to the general theory of descent—or apart from the more special problem of heredity—follow by way of logical consequence. In the latter case, there is no justification for any such deductions. For, no matter how faintly or how fitfully the hereditary qualities of the material in question may be modified by the somatic-tissues in which it resides, or by the external conditions of life to which it is exposed, these disturbances of its absolute stability, and these interruptions of its perpetual continuity, must cause more or less frequent changes on the part of its hereditary qualities—with the result that specific or other modifications of organic types need not have been solely due to the varying admixture of such material in sexual unions on the one hand, or to the unassisted power of natural selection on the other. Numberless additional causes of individual variation are admitted, while the Lamarckian principles are still allowed some degree of play. And although this is a lower degree than Darwin supposed, their influence in determining the course of organic evolution may still have been enormous; seeing that their action, in whatever measure it may be supposed to obtain, must always have been *cumulative* on the one hand, and *directive* of variations in adaptive lines on the other. Or, as Galton himself observes, in the passage already quoted, "if they exist, *in however faint a degree*, a complete theory of heredity must account for them." He saw, indeed, that a most inviting *logical* system could be framed by denying that they can ever exist in any degree—or, in other words, by supposing that stirp was *exactly* the same as what was afterwards called germ-plasm, in that it always occupied a separate "sphere" of its own, where its continuity has been uninterrupted "since the first origin of life." But Galton was not seduced by the temptation to construct an ideally logical system; and he had what I regard as the sound judgement to abstain from carrying his theory of stirp into any such transcendental "sphere" as that which is occupied by Weismann's theory of germ-plasm, in relation to the general doctrine of descent.

There is, then, a vast distinction between any theory of heredity which postulates the material of heredity as highly stable and largely continuous, and Weismann's theory,

33

which postulates this material as absolutely stable and perpetually continuous. But we must next take notice that Weismann himself has not kept this distinction in view with the constancy which we should have expected from so forcible a thinker. On the contrary, although in the construction of his theory of evolution he never fails to press the postulates of *absolute* stability and *perpetual* continuity to their logical conclusions in the various doctrines above enumerated (pp. 57-58), when engaged on his more special theory of heredity he every now and then appears to lose sight of the distinction. Indeed, he occasionally makes such large concessions with regard to both these postulates, that, were they to be entertained, the occupation of his critics would be gone: his theory of heredity would become converted into Galton's, while his theory of evolution would vanish altogether. It is therefore necessary to quote some of these concessions, if only to justify ourselves in subsequently ignoring them. I will give one instance of each; but it is necessary to preface the illustrations with a few words to mark emphatically three very distinct cases of congenital variation—leaving aside for the present the question whether or not they all occur in fact, as they are held to do by one or other of the theories of heredity.

1. The case where impoverished nutrition of the body has the effect of simply *starving* its germinal material. This is not a case where either the continuity or the stability of such material is affected. Its full efficiency as "formative material" may indeed be thus deteriorated to any extent, so that the progeny may be to any extent puny or malformed; but this will not necessarily cause any such re-shuffling of its "molecules" as will thereafter result in a permanent phylogenetic change. At most it will affect only the immediate offspring of poorly nourished parents; and natural selection will always be ready to eliminate such inefficient individuals. This case I will always hereafter call the case of *nutritive* congenital changes.

2. The case where germinal material is influenced by causes which do effect a re-shuffling of its "molecules," so that a permanent phylogenetic change does result. Observe, in this case, it does not signify whether the causes arise from external conditions of life, from any action of the soma on its own germinal material, or from so-called "spontaneous" changes on the part of such material itself. But the one cause which has not been concerned in producing an hereditary modification of this class is the mixture of "germ-plasms" in an act of sexual union. In hereafter speaking of this case I will follow Weismann's terminology, and call congenital changes thus produced *specialized* congenital changes.

3. Lastly, we have the case of the Lamarckian factors. This precisely resembles case 2, save that the congenital changes produced are still more "specialized." For while in the preceding case the re-shuffling before mentioned may have produced a congenital change of any kind, in the present case the congenital change produced must be of one particular kind—viz., a reproduction by heredity of the very same modification which occurred in the parents. "The fathers have eaten sour grapes, and the children's teeth are set on edge." This would be an extreme example of "use-inheritance," and so of case 3. But if the fathers had eaten sour grapes, and the children, instead of having their teeth set on edge, were to be born with a wryneck or a squint, then we should have a good example of case 2. In order, then, to mark the important distinction between these two cases, I will hereafter call the highly specialized changes due to the Lamarckian factors—supposing such changes to be possible—*representative* congenital changes.

34

These several distinctions being understood, I will proceed to furnish the two quotations from Weismann, which are respectively illustrative of his concessions touching his two fundamental postulates, as previously explained.

> We may fairly attribute to the adult organism influences which determine the phyletic development of its descendants. For the germ-cells are contained in the organism, and the external influences which affect them are intimately connected with the state of the organism in which they lie hid. If it be well nourished, the germ-cells will have abundant nutriment; and, conversely, if it be weak and sickly, the germ-cells will be arrested in their growth. It is even possible that the effects of these influences may be more specialized; that is to say, they may act only upon certain parts of the germ-cells. But this is indeed very different from believing that the changes of the organism which result from external stimuli can be transmitted to the germ-cells, and will re-develop in the next generation at the same time as that at which they arose in the parent, and in the same part of the organism[18].

It will be perceived that Weismann himself here very clearly draws all the distinctions between cases 1, 2, and 3, as above explained. Therefore it becomes the more remarkable that he should not have perceived how radically inconsistent it is in him thus to entertain as "possible" congenital variations belonging to the case 2. For, as we have now so fully seen, the theory of germ-plasm (as distinguished from that of stirp) cannot entertain the possibility of an hereditary and specialized change of *any* kind as thus produced by external conditions of life: should such a possibility be entertained, there must obviously be an end to the *absolute stability* of germ-plasm, and a consequent collapse of Weismann's theory of evolution. Either germ-plasm is absolutely stable, or else it is but highly stable. If it is absolutely stable, individual variations of an hereditary kind can occur only as results of sexual admixtures of germ-plasm, and Weismann's theory of evolution is established. But if germ-plasm is not absolutely stable (no matter in how high a degree it may be so) hereditary individual variations may be produced by other causes, and Weismann's theory of evolution collapses. Therefore, if we are to examine his theory of *evolution*, we can do so only by ignoring such a passage as the one just quoted, which surrenders the postulate of the *absolute stability* of germ-plasm.

Again, if we are to examine Weismann's theory of *heredity*, we must similarly ignore such a passage as the following, where he represents that he is similarly prepared to surrender his still more fundamental postulate of the *perpetual continuity* of germ-plasm.

After remarking that some of his own experiments on the climatic varieties of certain butterflies raise such difficulties against his whole theory of heredity that even now "he cannot explain the facts otherwise than by supposing the passive acquisition of characters produced by the direct influence of climate," he goes on to remark more generally—"We cannot exclude the possibility of such a transmission occasionally occurring, for, even if the greater part of the effects must be attributed to natural selection, there might be a smaller part in certain cases which depends on this exceptional factor[19]"—i.e., the Lamarckian factor!

Now, it must be particularly noted that in this passage Weismann is speaking, not as in the previous passage, of *specialized* congenital characters, but of *representative* congenital characters. In other words, he here entertains the possibility which in the passage previously quoted he very properly rejects—namely, "that changes of the organism which result from external stimuli can be transmitted to the germ-cells, and will re-develop in the next generation *at the same time as that at which they arose in the parent, and in the same part of the organism*." But it is evident that if the theory of germ-plasm is undermined by the concession made in the passage thus previously quoted, in the passage last quoted a match is put to the fuse. It does not signify whether the particular case of the butterflies in question will ever admit of any other explanation more in accordance with the theory of germ-plasm: the point is that in *no* case can this theory entertain the possibility of causes other than admixtures of germ-plasm in sexual unions producing hereditary changes, (A) of *any* kind, (B) still less of a *specialized* kind, and (C) least of all of a *representative* kind. For the distinguishing essence of this theory is, that germ-plasm must always have moved, so to speak, in a closed orbit of its own: its "sphere" must have been perpetually distinct from those of whatever other "plasms" there may be in the constellations of living things. So that, in such passages as those just quoted, Weismann is not only destroying the very foundations of his general theory of evolution, but at the same time he is identifying his more special theory of heredity with those which had been already published by his predecessors, and more particularly by Galton. Now, it is not Galton's theory that we are considering; and therefore we must hereafter ignore those fundamental admissions, whereby Weismann every now and again appears ready to relinquish all that is most distinctive of, or original in, his own elaborate system of theories.

It is, indeed, impossible not to admire the candour of these admissions, or to avoid recognizing the truly scientific spirit which they betoken. But, at the same time, one is led to doubt whether in making them Professor Weismann has sufficiently considered their full import. He appears to deem it of comparatively little importance whether or not acquired characters can sometimes and in some degrees influence the hereditary qualities of germ-plasm, provided he can show that *much the larger* part of the phenomena of heredity must be ascribed to the continuity of germ-plasm. In other words, he seems to think that it matters but little whether in the course of organic evolution the Lamarckian factors have played but a very subordinate part, or whether they have not played any part at all. Moreover, I have heard one or two prominent followers of Weismann give public expression to the same opinion. Therefore I must repeat that it makes a literally immeasurable difference whether we suppose, with Galton, that the Lamarckian factors may sometimes and in some degrees assert themselves, or whether we suppose, with the great bulk of Weismann's writings and in accordance with the logical requirements of *his* theory, that they can never possibly occur in any degree. The distinctive postulate of his theory of heredity, and one of the two fundamental doctrines on which he founds his further theory of evolution, is, that the physiology of sexual reproduction cannot admit of any inversion of the relations between "germ-plasm" and "somatic idio-plasm[20]." This is a perfectly intelligible postulate, but it is not one with which we may play fast and loose. Either there is such a physiological mechanism as it announces, in which case the relations in question can never be inverted "occasionally," any more than rags may "occasionally" help to construct the mill which is to form them into paper;—or else there is no such mechanism, in which case we may have to do with gemmules, physiological units, stirp, micellae, pangenes, plastidules, or any of the other hypothetical "carriers of heredity" to which our predilections may happen to incline; but the one substance with which we certainly have not to do is germ-plasm[21].

36

After these tedious but necessary preambles, we may now proceed to examine Professor Weismann's postulate as to the perpetual continuity of germ-plasm, with its superstructure in his theory of heredity—reserving for the next chapter our examination of his further postulate touching the absolute stability of germ-plasm, with its superstructure in his theory of evolution.

The evidence which Weismann has presented in favour of his fundamental postulate of the perpetual continuity of germ-plasm may be conveniently dealt with under two heads—namely, indirect evidence as derived from general reasoning, and direct evidence derived from particular facts.

The general reasoning is directed to show, (1) that there is no evidence of the transmission of acquired characters; (2) that the theory of pangenesis is "inconceivable"; and, (3) that the alternative theory of germ-plasm is amply conceivable. Now, to the best of my judgement, not one of these propositions is borne out by the general reasoning in question. But as the latter is almost entirely of an *a priori* character, and also of a somewhat abstruse construction, I think the patience of any ordinary reader will be saved by relegating this part of our subject to an Appendix. Therefore, remarking only that any one who cares to look at Appendix I ought, in my opinion, to perceive that there is no real evidence against the transmission of acquired characters to be derived from Weismann's general reasoning in this connexion, I will at once proceed to consider the evidence which he has adduced in the way of particular facts.

In the first place, as one result of his brilliant researches on the *Hydromedusae*, he has found that the generative cells occur only in certain localized situations, which, however, vary greatly in different species, though they are always constant for the same species. He also found that the varying situations in different species of the localized or generative areas correspond, place for place, with successive stages in a process of gradual transposition which has occurred in the phylogeny of the *Hydromedusae*. Lastly, he has found that in each ontogeny these successive stages of transposition are repeated, with the result that during the individual lifetime of one of these animals the germ-cells migrate through the body, from what used to be their ancestral situation to what is now the normal situation for that particular species. Such being the facts, Weismann argues from them that the germ-cells of the *Hydromedusae* are thus proved to present properties of a peculiar kind, which cannot be supplied by any of the other cells of the organism; for, if they could, whence the necessity for this migration of these particular cells? Of course it follows that these peculiar properties must depend on the presence of some peculiar substance, and that this is none other than the "germ-plasm," which here exhibits a demonstrable "continuity" throughout the entire phylogeny of these unquestionably very ancient Metazoa.

The second line of direct evidence in favour of the continuity of germ-plasm which Weismann has adduced is, that in the case of some invertebrated animals the sexual apparatus is demonstrably separated as reproductive cells (or cells which afterwards give rise to the reproductive glands) at a very early period of ontogeny—so early indeed, in certain cases, that this separation constitutes actually the first stage in the process of ontogeny. Therefore, it is argued, we may regard it as antecedently improbable that the after-life of the individual can in any way affect the congenital endowments of its ova, seeing that the ova have been thus from the first anatomically isolated from all the other tissues of the organism.

The third and only other line of direct evidence is, that organisms which have been produced parthenogenetically, or without admixture of germ-plasms in any previous act of sexual fertilization, do not exhibit congenital variations.

Taking, then, these three lines of verification separately, none of them need detain us long. For although the fact of the migration of germ-cells becomes one of great interest in relation to Weismann's theory *after the theory has been accepted*, the fact in itself does not furnish any evidence in support of the theory. In the first place, it tends equally well to support Galton's theory of stirp; and therefore does not lend any special countenance to the theory of germ-plasm—or the theory that there cannot now be, and never can have been, any communication at all between the plasm of the germ and that of the soma. In the second place, the fact of such migration is not incompatible even with the theory of pangenesis, or the theory which supposes such a communication to be extremely intimate. There may be many other reasons for this migration of germ-cells besides the one which Weismann's theory supposes. For example, the principle of physiological economy may very well have determined that it is better to continue for reproductive purposes the use of cells which have already been specialized and set apart for the execution of those purposes, than to discard these cells and transform others into a kind fitted to replace them. Even the theory of pangenesis requires to assume a very high degree of specialization on the part of germ-cells; and as it is the fact of such specialization alone which is proved by Weismann's observations, I do not see that it constitutes any criterion between his theory of heredity and that of Darwin—still less, of course, between his theory and that of Galton. Lastly, in this connexion we ought to remember that the *Hydromedusae* are organisms in which the specialization in question happens to be least, as is shown by the fact that entire individuals admit of being reproduced from fragments of somatic-tissues; so that these are organisms where we would least expect to meet with the migration of germ-cells, were the purpose of such migration that which Weismann suggests. This line of evidence therefore seems valueless.

Nor does it appear to me that the second line of evidence is of any more value. In the first place, there is no shadow of a reason for supposing that an apparently anatomical isolation of germ-cells necessarily entails a physiological isolation as regards their special function—all "physiological analogy," indeed, being opposed to such a view, as is shown in Appendix I. In the second place, there is no proof of any anatomical isolation, as we may likewise see in that Appendix. In the third place, the fact relied upon to indicate such an isolation—viz., the early formation of germ-cells—is not a fact of any general occurrence. On the contrary, it obtains only in a comparatively small number of animals, while it does not obtain in any plants. In the Vertebrates, for example, the reproductive cells are not differentiated from the somatic cells till after the embryo has been fully formed; while in plants their development constitutes the very last stage of ontogeny. In the fourth place, the argument, even for what it is worth, is purely deductive; and deductive reasoning in such a case as this—where the phenomena are enormously complex and our ignorance unusually profound—is always precarious. Lastly, in the fifth place, Weismann has now himself abandoned this argument. For in one of his later essays he says:—

> Those instances of early separation of sexual from somatic cells, upon which I have often insisted as indicating the continuity of the germ-plasm, do not now appear to be of such conclusive importance as at the time when we were not sure

about the localization of the plasm in the nuclei. In the great majority of cases the germ-cells are not separated at the beginning of embryonic development, but only in some of the later stages.... It therefore follows that cases of early separation of the germ-cells afford no proof of a direct persistence of the parent germ-cells in those of the offspring.

The last line of direct evidence, or that derived from the alleged non-variability of parthenogenetic organisms, is, as Professor Vines has shown, opposed to fact. Therefore, in his later writings, Weismann has abandoned this line of evidence also.

Upon the whole,then, we must conclude with regard to the fundamental postulate of perpetual continuity, that there is actually no evidence of a direct kind in its favour. And, as Weismann's arguments of an indirect kind are dealt with in Appendix I, it remains only to state such evidence *per contra* as, to the best of my judgement, appears valid.

The fundamental proposition which we have been considering, and to the further consideration of which we have now to proceed, is, in effect, that germ-plasm differs from stirp in having been *perpetually* restricted to a "sphere" of its own, "*since the first origin of life.*" Criticism, therefore, must be directed to show that the "sphere" in question has not been proved so entirely independent as this fundamental proposition sets forth; but that, on the contrary, there appears to be a certain amount of reciprocal action between this sphere and that of the somatic-tissues—even though we may agree (as I myself agree) with Galton in holding that the degree of such reciprocal action is neither so intimate nor so constant as it was held to be by Darwin. This, indeed, is the direction which the course of our criticism has taken already. For it has just been shown that Weismann has failed to adduce any facts (preceding text) or considerations (Appendix I) in support of his fundamental proposition as above stated, save such as proceed on a prior acceptance of the proposition itself. The facts and considerations which he has adduced are therefore useless as evidence in support of this proposition, although they would admit of being explained by it supposing it to have been already substantiated by any facts or considerations of an independent kind. Which is merely another way of saying, as already said, that there is no evidence in favour of the proposition.

But I am now about to argue that there *is* evidence *against* the proposition. For I am about to argue, not only as heretofore that for anything Weismann has shown to the contrary there *may* be a certain amount of reciprocal action between the sphere of germinal-substance and the sphere of body-substance; but that, as a matter of fact, there *is* a certain amount of such reciprocal action.

Without laying undue stress on the intimate "correlation" that subsists between the reproductive organs and all other parts of the organism, I nevertheless think that the fact ought here to be noted. For the changes which occur at puberty and after the reproductive functions have ceased, as well as those which may be artificially produced by castration, &c., prove at any rate some extremely important association between the soma as a whole and its reproductive apparatus as a whole. No doubt it may properly enough be answered that this proof does not extend to the vital point of showing the association to be between the soma as a whole, and that particular part of the reproductive apparatus in which the "carriers of heredity" reside—namely, the ova and spermatozoa; and, therefore, that the facts in question may be due only to some changed conditions of nutrition on the part of the somatic-tissues which these alterations on the part of the reproductive glands entail. On this account we must fully allow that the facts in question are not in themselves of any conclusive weight; but I think they are worth mentioning, because they certainly seem to countenance the theory which supposes some reciprocal influence as exercised by the germinal elements on the somatic-tissues and *vice versa*, rather than they do the theory which supposes the germinal elements and the somatic-tissues to have always occupied totally different "spheres."

Here, however, is a stronger class of facts. It has not unfrequently been observed, at any rate in mammals, that when a female has borne progeny to a male of one variety, and subsequently bears progeny to a male of another variety, the younger progeny presents a more or less unmistakable resemblance to the father of the older one. Now, this is a fact to which Weismann has nowhere alluded; and therefore I do not know how he would meet it. But, as far as I can see, it can be explained only in one or other of two ways. Either there must be some action of the spermatic element on the hitherto unripe ovum, or else this element must exercise some influence on the somatic-tissues of the female, which in their turn act upon the ovum[22]. Now, I do not deny that the first of these possibilities might be reconcilable with the hypothesis of an absolute continuity of germ-plasm; for it is conceivable that the life of germ-plasm is not coterminous with that of the spermatozoa which convey it, and hence that, if the carriers of heredity, after the disintegration of their containing spermatozoa, should ever penetrate an unripe ovum, the germ-plasm thus introduced might remain dormant in the ovum until the latter becomes mature, and is then fertilized by another sire. In this way it is conceivable that the hitherto dormant germ-plasm of the previous sire might exercise some influence on the progeny of a subsequent one. But it seems clear that the second of the two possibilities above named could not be thus brought within the hypothesis of an absolute continuity of germ-plasm. Therefore it seems that the school of Weismann must adopt the first, to the exclusion of the second. Unfortunately for them, however, there is another (and clearly analogous) fact, which goes to exclude the first possibility, and most definitely to substantiate the second. For, in the case of plants, where there can be no second progeny borne by the same "ovary," but where we happen to be able to see that a marked effect is sometimes produced on the somatic-tissues of the mother by the pollen of the father, there can be no question as to the male element being able to exercise a direct influence on the soma of the female. Consequently, whatever we may think with regard to the case of animals, the facts with regard to plants are in themselves enough to sustain the only position with which we are concerned—viz., that the male element is capable of directly modifying the female soma.

The facts with regard to plants are these. When one variety fertilizes the ovules of another, not unfrequently the influence extends beyond the ovules to the ovarium, and even to the calyx and flower-stalk, of the mother plant. This influence, which may affect the shape, size, colour, and texture of the somatic-tissues of the mother, has been observed in a large number of plants belonging to many different orders. The details of the matter have already been dealt with by Darwin, in the eleventh chapter of his work on *Variation*, &c.; and this is what he says. The italics are mine.

> The proofs of the action of foreign pollen on the mother-plant have been given in considerable detail, because this action is of the highest theoretical importance, and because it is in itself a remarkable and apparently anomalous circumstance. That it is remarkable under a physiological point of view is clear, for the male element not only affects, in accordance with its proper function, the germ, but at the same time various parts of the mother-plant, *in the same manner as it affects*

the same parts in the seminal offspring from the same two parents. We thus learn that an ovule is not indispensable for the reception of the influence of the male element.

Darwin then proceeds to show that this direct action of the male element on the somatic tissues of another organism is not so rare or anomalous as it at first sight appears; for in the case of not a few flowers it comes into play as a needful preliminary to fertilization. Thus, for instance:—

> Gärtner gradually increased the number of pollen grains until he succeeded in fertilizing a Malva, and has proved that many grains are first expended in the development, or, as he expresses it, in the satiation, of the pistil and ovarium. Again, when one plant is fertilized by a widely distinct species, it often happens that the ovarium is fully and quickly developed without any seeds being formed; or the coats of the seeds are formed without any embryo being developed therein.

So much, then, in proof of the direct action of the male element on the somatic-tissues of another organism. It remains to show that a similar action may be exercised by this element on the somatic tissues of its own organism. This has been proved by Hildebrand, who found "that in the normal fertilization of several Orchideae, the action of the plant's own pollen is necessary for the development of the ovarium; and that this development takes place not only long before the pollen tubes have reached the ovules, but even before the placentae and ovules have been formed"; so that with these orchids the pollen acts directly on their own ovaria, as a preliminary to the formation of the ovules which are subsequently to be fertilized.

It is to be regretted that Professor Weismann has not given us his opinion upon this whole class of facts, for assuredly they appear directly to contradict his theory. The theory is, "that the germ-plasm and the somato-plasm have always occupied different spheres": the fact is, that the germ-plasm may directly act upon the somato-plasm, both within and beyond the limits of the same organism.

Hitherto we have been considering certain very definite facts, which seem to prove that the germinal elements are able directly to affect the somatic-tissues. We have next to consider such facts as seem to prove the opposite side of a reciprocal relationship— viz., that the somatic-tissues are able directly to affect the germinal elements.

And here there are two distinct lines of evidence to be distinguished.

Firstly, in certain cases—exceptional it is true, but this does not signify—somatic-tissues have been found capable of modifying the hereditary endowments of germinal elements by means of simple grafting. This line of evidence has also been disregarded both by Weismann and his followers; but it is nevertheless an important one to consider. For, if it be the case that the somatic-tissues of an organism A, by being merely grafted on-those of organism B, can so affect the germinal elements of B as to cause their offspring to resemble A—or, contrariwise, if the somatic-tissues of A can thus act on B—then, although it may not be properly said that any "acquired characters" have been transmitted from A to the progeny of B, (or *vice versa*,) such an a-sexual transmission of alien characters, in its relation to the theory of germ-plasm, is scarcely less awkward than are certain facts which they appear to prove.

Secondly, that acquired characters may be transmitted to progeny by the more ordinary methods of sexual propagation (Lamarckian factors). This second line of evidence will be fully and independently dealt with in future chapters, specially devoted to the subject. Therefore we have here to consider only the first.

Now, the force of this first line of evidence will become apparent, if we reflect that the only way in which the facts can be met by Weismann's theory, would be by supposing that the somatic germ-plasms which are respectively diffused through the cellular tissues of the scion and the graft become mixed in some such way as they might have been, had the hybrid been due to seminal propagation instead of to simple grafting. But against this, the only interpretation of the facts which is open to the theory, there lies the following objection, which to me appears insuperable.

Where sexual cells are concerned there is always a definite arrangement to secure penetration of the one by the other, and we can see the necessity for such an arrangement in order to effect an admixture of their nuclear contents, where alone germ-plasm is supposed by Weismann's theory to reside. But in tissue-cells, which have not been thus specialized, it would be difficult to believe that nuclear contents can admit of being intimately fused by a mere apposition of cell-walls. For not only are the nuclear contents of any two such cells thus separated from one another by two cell-walls and two masses of "cytoplasm"; but it is not enough to suppose that in order to produce a graft-hybrid only two of these somatic-cells need mix their nuclear contents, as we know is all that is required in order to produce a seminal hybrid by means of sexual cells. On the contrary, in the former case most, if not all, the somatic-cells which are brought into apposition by the graft must be supposed thus to mix their nuclear contents at the plane of the graft; for otherwise the hybrid would not afterwards present equally the characters of stock and scion. Now, there may be hundreds of thousands of such cells, and therefore it seems impossible that the facts of graft-hybridization can be reconciled with the theory of germ-plasms[23].

The third line of evidence against this theory—i.e., the evidence in favour of the transmission of acquired characters—is to constitute the subject-matter of future chapters. Therefore it will here be sufficient to adduce only one fact of this kind. And I select it because it is one that has been dealt with by Weismann himself. In one of his more recent statements he says:—

> The distinguished botanist De Vries has proved that certain constituents of the cell body—e. g., the chromatophores of Algae—pass directly from the maternal ovum to the daughter organism, while the male germ-cells generally contain no chromatophores. Here it appears possible that a transmission of somatogenetic variation has occurred[24].

Now although, as Weismann goes on to observe, "in these lower plants, the separation between somatic and reproductive cells is slight," in the facts to which he alludes we appear to have good evidence of an influence exercised by somatic cells upon the germinal contents of reproductive cells. And if such an influence is capable of being exercised in the case of "these lower plants," it follows that there is no such *absolute* separation between somatic tissues and germ-plasm as Weismann's theory requires. Moreover it follows that, if the essential distinction between germ-plasm and somato-plasm (or "somatic idio-plasm") is thus violated at the very foundation of the multicellular organisms, there ceases to be any *a priori* reason for drawing arbitrary limits, either as to the level of organization at which such "transmission of somatogenetic variation has occurred," or as to the degree of detail into which it may extend. Both these matters then stand to be tested by observation; and the burden of proof lies with the school of Weismann to show at what level of organization, and at what degree of representation, somatogenetic changes cease to reproduce themselves by heredity.

Passing on, then, to higher levels of organization, and therefore to higher degrees of representation, I shall endeavour to show that this burden of proof cannot be discharged. For I shall endeavour to show, not merely, as just shown, that there ceases to be any *a priori* reason for drawing arbitrary limits with respect either to levels of organization or to degrees of representation, but that, as a matter of fact, there are no such limits as the passage above quoted assigns. On the contrary, I believe there is as good evidence to prove the not unfrequent transmission of acquired ("somatogenetic") characters among the higher plants—and even among the higher animals—as there is of the occurrence of this phenomenon in the case of the Alga just mentioned. But in order to do this evidence justice, I shall have to take a new point of departure and consider as a separate question the transmissibility of acquired characters. Meanwhile, and as far as Weismann's theory of heredity is concerned, it is enough to have shown,—if I have been successful in doing so,—that not only is there no evidence to sustain his fundamental postulate touching the material of heredity having always occupied a separate "sphere" of its own "since the first origin of life"; but that there is good evidence to prove the contrary. For whether or not the reciprocal action of "somato-plasm" and "germ-plasm" can ever proceed to the extent of causing acquired characters to be inherited (so as to produce "representative congenital changes"), all that is distinctive in this theory must be regarded as barren speculation, unless it can be shown that the foregoing facts have failed to prove such a reciprocal action as ever occurring in any lower degree (so as to produce "specialized congenital changes").

CHAPTER IV.

EXAMINATION OF WEISMANN'S THEORY OF EVOLUTION (1891).

HAVING now considered germ-plasm as perpetually continuous, we have next to regard it as unalterably stable.

First, let it be noted that these two fundamental and distinctive postulates of the whole Weismannian system are so intimately connected as to be in large measure mutually dependent. For, on the one hand, if germ-plasm has not been perpetually continuous since the first origin of life, it cannot have been absolutely stable "since the first origin of sexual propagation": every time that its hereditary characters are modified by its containing soma (whether or not representatively so), its stability has been so far upset. On the other hand, if germ-plasm has not been absolutely stable, it cannot have been perpetually continuous "since the first origin of life." As often as its stability has been upset, its "molecular structure" has been modified by causes *ab extra*, as distinguished from mixtures of germ-plasms in sexual unions. Therefore, it can no longer have been continuous in the sense of having borne an ineffaceable record of all congenital variations, *due to sexual unions*, throughout the entire phylogeny of the Metaphyta and Metazoa. At most it can have been continuous only in the attenuated sense, that however much and however often its hereditary characters may have been modified by somatic changes on the one hand or by changes in the external conditions of life on the other, they can never have been thus modified *representatively*, as supposed by the theory of pangenesis.

From which it follows that, while examining in our last chapter Weismann's doctrine of the perpetual continuity of germ-plasm, we have been indirectly examining also his companion doctrine of the unalterable stability of germ-plasm. Nevertheless, for the sake of doing justice to both these doctrines, I have thought it desirable to examine each on its own merits, without prejudice arising from our criticism of the other. To such a separate and independent examination of the doctrine of unalterable stability we will, therefore, now proceed.

As we have already and repeatedly seen, this doctrine of the unalterable or absolute stability of germ-plasm "since the first origin of sexual propagation" is a logically essential part of Weismann's theory of evolution, or of his system of hypotheses considered as a whole. It is so because upon this doctrine depends his reference of individual variations in the Metazoa to an ultimate origin in the Protozoa, the significance of sexual reproduction in the theory of natural selection, &c., &c. Therefore this doctrine of the absolute stability of germ-plasm is enunciated by Weismann, not merely for the purpose of meeting any one class of facts, such as those of atavism, persistence of rudimentary organs, &c. The doctrine is enunciated for the purpose of constituting one of the foundation-stones of his general theory of evolution. We have now to consider how far the quality of this stone renders it trustworthy as a basis to build upon.

In the first place, we can scarcely fail to perceive that this doctrine of the absolute stability of germ-plasm is not only gratuitous, but intrinsically improbable. That the most complex material in nature should likewise be the most stable is opposed to all the analogies of nature, and therefore to all the probabilities of the case.

Again, the germ-plasm, as it originally occurred (and still exists) in unicellular organisms, is supposed to be exactly the same *kind* of material as now occurs in the germ-cells of multicellular organisms. Yet the very same theory which supposes so absolute a stability on the part of germ-plasm when located in germ-cells (or diffused through somatic-cells), likewise supposes so high a degree of variability on the part of germ-plasm when not thus located, as to represent that all individual variations which have ever taken place in the unicellular organisms—and all the innumerable species of such organisms which have arisen therefrom—have been due to the direct action of external conditions of life; or, in other words, to the *instability* of germ-plasm. The very same substance which at one time and in one place is supposed to be so absolutely unchangeable, at another time and in another place is supposed to be highly susceptible of change.

Lastly—and this is, perhaps, the most curious part of the whole matter—the place where germ-plasm is supposed to be unchangeable is not the place where it is most likely to be so, but the place where it is least likely. For germ-plasm as it occurs in the germ-cells of multicellular organisms must have a constitution greatly more complex even than that which it has in unicellular organisms—seeing that in the former case, and by hypothesis, it bears a living record of the whole phylogeny of the Metaphyta and Metazoa in all their innumerable branchings. And not only so, but when germ-plasm occurs in germ-cells it becomes exposed to much greater vicissitudes: its environment has become vastly more complex, as well as greatly more liable to change with the changing conditions of life of the many mutable species in which it resides, and on the individual somas of which it now depends for its nourishment. So that, altogether, we have here on merely *a priori* grounds about as strong a case against this doctrine of absolute stability as it is well conceivable that on merely *a priori* grounds a case can be.

Turning next to arguments *a posteriori*, let us begin by considering those which Weismann has adduced in support of the doctrine.

First, he alleges that there is a total absence of variability on the part of all organisms which have been produced parthenogenetically, or from unfertilized ova. We may look in vain, he says, for any individual differences on the part of any multicellular organisms, which have been brought into existence independently of the blending of germ-plasms in a previous act of sexual union. Now, unquestionably, if this statement could be corroborated by sufficiently extensive observation, the fact would become one of immense significance—so much so, indeed, that of itself it would go far to neutralize all antecedent objections, and to verify his theory as to sexual propagation being the sole cause of congenital variation. But seeing that the alleged fact stands so entirely out of analogy with the phenomena of bud-variation (which will be alluded to later on), it is highly improbable, even on antecedent grounds; while Professor Vines has refuted the statement on grounds of actual fact. Thus, speaking of the *Basidiomycetes*, he says—

> These Fungi are not only entirely a-sexual, but it would appear that they have been evolved in a purely a-sexual manner from a-sexual ascomycetous or æcidiomycetous ancestors. The Basidiomycetes, in fact, afford an example of a vast family of plants, of the most varied form and habit, including hundreds of genera and species, in which, so far as minute and long-continued investigation has shown, there is not, and probably never has been, any trace of a sexual process[25].

Here, then, we have actual proof of "hereditary individual variations" among a-sexually propagating organisms, sufficient in amount to have given origin, not merely to "individual differences," but to innumerable species, and even genera. Consequently Weismann allows that the criticism abolishes this line of evidence in favour of the absolute stability of germ-plasm[26]. Consquently, also, we must now add, in whatever measure the alleged fact would have corroborated the theory had it been proved to be a fact, in that measure is the theory discredited by proof that it is not a fact. For, if the theory were sound, this particular fact would certainly have admitted of demonstration: therefore the proof that it is not a fact—but the reverse of a fact—amounts at the same time to a disproof of the theory[27].

The only other line of evidence to be adduced in favour of the absolute stability of germ-plasm is that which is furnished by the high antiquity of some specific types, by the facts of atavism, and by the persistency of vestigial organs. But this line of evidence is as futile as the other. Nobody has ever questioned that hereditary characters are persistently stable as long as they are persistently maintained by natural selection; and this, according to Weismann himself, must have been the case with all long-enduring species: these, therefore, fail to furnish any evidence of the *inherent* stability of germ-plasm, which is the only point in question.

Again, as regards the facts of atavism, nobody is disputing these facts. What we are disputing is whether the *degree* of inherent stability which they unquestionably prove can be rationally regarded as such that it may endure, not merely for such a comparatively small number of generations as these facts imply, but actually for any number of generations, or through the practically infinite series of generations that now intervene between the higher metazoa and their primeval parentage in the protozoa. Clearly, the ratio between these two things is such that no argument derived from the facts of atavism can be of any avail for the purposes of this Weismannian doctrine.

Lastly, as regards vestigial organs, the consideration that, surprisingly persistent as they unquestionably are, nevertheless they do eventually disappear, seems to prove that the power of heredity does in time become exhausted, even in cases most favourable to its continuance. That it should thus become finally exhausted is no more than Darwin's theory of perishable gemmules, or Galton's theory of a not absolutely stable stirp, would expect. But the fact is irreconcilable with Weismann's theory of an absolutely stable germ-plasm.

Hence, we can only conclude that there is no evidence in favour of the hypothesis that germ-plasm has been unalterably stable "since the first origin of sexual propagation"; while the suggestion that it may have been so is on antecedent grounds improbable, and on inductive grounds untenable. It only remains to add that the *degree* of stability has been proved in not a few cases to be less than even the theory of gemmules might anticipate. Many facts in proof of this statement might be given, but it will here suffice to quote one, which I select because it has been dealt with by Professor Weismann himself.

Professor Hoffmann has published an abstract of a research, which consisted in subjecting plants with normal flowers to changed conditions of life through a series of generations. In course of time, certain well-marked variations appeared. Now, in some cases such directly-produced variations were transmitted by seed from the affected plants; and therefore Weismann acknowledges,—"I have no doubt that the results are, at any rate in part, due to the operation of heredity." Hence, whether these results be due to the transmission of somatogenetic characters ("representative changes"), or to the direct action of changed conditions of life on the germ-plasm itself ("specialized changes"), it is equally certain that the hereditary characters of the plants were congenitally modified to a large extent, within (at most) a few generations. In other words, it is certain that, if there be such a material as germ-plasm, it has been proved in this case to have been highly unstable. Therefore, in dealing with these and other similar facts, Weismann himself can only save his postulate of continuity by surrendering for the time being his postulate of stability[28].

If to this it be replied that Hoffmann's facts are exceptional—that Gärtner, Nägeli, De Candolle, Peter, Jordan, and others, did not find individual variations produced in plants by changed conditions of life to be inherited,—the reply would be irrelevant. It does not require to be proved that all variations produced by changed conditions of life are inherited. If only some—even though it be but an extremely small percentage—of such variations are proved to be inherited, the many millions of years that separate the germ-plasm of to-day from its supposed origin in the protozoa, must have furnished opportunities enough for the occurrence of such variations to have obliterated, and re-obliterated numberless times, any aboriginal differences in the germ-plasms of incipiently sexual organisms. Moreover, it is probable that when further experiments shall have been made in this direction, Hoffmann's results will be found not so exceptional as they at present appear. Mr. Mivart, for example, has mentioned several instances[29]; while there are not a few facts of general knowledge—such as the modifications undergone by certain Crustacea as a direct result of increased salinity of the water in which they live—that will probably soon be proved to be facts of the same order. But here attention must be directed to another large body of facts, which are of high importance in the present connexion.

The phenomena of what is called bud-variation in plants are phenomena of not infrequent occurrence, and they consist in the sudden appearance of a peculiarity on the part of a shoot which develops from a single bud. When such a peculiarity arises, it admits of being propagated, not only by cuttings and by other buds from that shoot, but sometimes also by seeds which the flowers of the shoot subsequently produce—in which case all the laws of inheritance that apply to congenital variations are found to apply also to bud-variation. Or, as Darwin puts it, "there is not any particular in which new characters arising by bud-variation can be distinguished from those due to seminal variation"; and, therefore, any theory which deals with the latter is bound also to take cognizance of the former. Now, as far as I can find, there is only one paragraph in which Weismann alludes to bud-variation, and what he there says I do not find very easy to understand. Therefore I will quote the whole paragraph *verbatim*.

> I have not hitherto considered budding in relation to my theories, but it is obvious that it is to be explained, from my point of view, by supposing that the germ-plasm which passes on into a budding individual consists not only of the unchanged germ-plasm of the first ontogenetic stage, but of this substance altered, so far as to correspond with the altered structure of the individual which arises from it—viz., the rootless shoot which springs from the stem or branches. The alteration must be very slight, and perhaps quite insignificant, for it is possible that the differences between the secondary shoots and the primary plant may depend chiefly on the changed conditions of development, which takes place beneath the earth in the latter case, and in the tissues of the plant in the former. Thus we may imagine that the idio-plasm [? of that particular bud], when it develops into a flowering shoot, produces at the same time the germ-cells which are found in the latter. We thus approach an understanding of Fritz Müller's observation; for if the whole shoot which produces the flower arises from the same idio-plasm which also forms its germ-cells, we can readily understand why the latter should contain the same hereditary tendencies which were previously expressed in the flower which produced them. The fact that variations may occur in a single shoot depends on the changes explained above, which occur in the idio-plasm during the course of its growth, as a result of the varying proportions in which the ancestral idio-plasms may be contained in it.[30]

The meaning here appears to be twofold. For there are only two ways of explaining the phenomena of bud-variation. Either they are due to the influence of external conditions acting on the particular bud in question, or else they are due to so-called "spontaneous" changes taking place within the bud itself. Possibly it may be both, but at least it must be either. Well, in the above passage, Weismann appears to assume that it is both. For at the beginning of the passage he speaks of the "germ-plasm of the first ontogenetic stage" becoming "altered so far as to correspond with the altered structure of the individual which arises therefrom," and he goes on to say that the alteration "may depend chiefly on the changed conditions of development"—that is, as I understand, the influence of external conditions. But at the end of the paragraph he says that "the changes which occur in the idio-plasm during the course of its growth" in the sporting bud, are due to "the varying proportions in which the ancestral idio-plasms may be contained in it." Thus, I take it, Weismann here entertains both explanations of the phenomena in question: he appears to regard these phenomena as partly due to peculiar admixtures of ancestral idio-plasms in the bud itself (or "spontaneous" variation), but partly also to an alteration of the germ-plasm by its changed condition of development (or variation caused by external conditions).

However, it is but of little consequence whether or not this is the meaning which Weismann intends to convey. For the point we are coming to is, that, whatever he intends to convey, "from the point of view" of the theory of germ-plasm, there is only *one* interpretation possible. It is not open to Weismann (as it was to Darwin, or even to Galton,) to entertain *both* the explanations, whether separately or in conjunction. For germ-plasm (unlike gemmules, or even stirp) must be held always and everywhere *unalterably* stable: else the whole superstructure of Weismann's theory of evolution falls to the ground. We cannot consent to his retaining this theory on the one hand, and, on the other, explaining bud-variation by "germ-plasm of the first ontogenetic stage" becoming altered "chiefly by changed conditions of development." Even if it were true that "the alteration must be very slight, if not quite insignificant," there would here be a rift in the lute, which must finally stop any further harping on the subject of Evolution.

From the point of view of this theory, then, there is only one interpretation open,—viz., that a bud-variation is ultimately due to a peculiar admixture of germ-plasms in the seed from which the bud was ultimately derived. But the objections to entertaining this as even a logically possible explanation of the phenomena in all cases, is insuperable.

In the first place, such a variation, when it does arise, is usually a variation of an extremely pronounced character; therefore it is very far from supporting Weismann's view, that the "alteration" of germ-plasm which is needed to produce it "must be very slight, and perhaps quite insignificant." In most cases where it occurs bud-variation presents so extreme a departure from the normal type, that no other kind of variation can be fitly compared with it in this respect. In particular, the degree of variation is usually very much greater than that which customarily obtains in congenital variations of the ordinary kind; and, therefore, if these be supposed due to particular admixtures of germ-plasm in sexual propagation, much more must those admixtures which give rise to sporting buds be characterized by peculiarities of no "insignificant" order. And much more, therefore, ought they to assert themselves in sister-buds developed from the same individual seed (ovule), than we find to be the case with any sister-organisms which are developed from different individual seeds. Yet, in the second place, so far is this from being the case, that the most remarkable feature connected with bud-variation—next to the suddenness and extreme amount of the variation itself—is the usually isolated nature of its occurrence. There may be thousands of other buds on the same plant, and yet it is one bud alone that deviates so suddenly and so widely from its ancestral characters. Nay, more, a single bud-variation may—and usually does—occur in plants which are habitually propagated by cuttings and graftings; so that there may not only be thousands, but millions of buds all derived from one original seed, and all for many years remaining perfectly true to their parent type, with the single exception of the sporting bud, which, while it departs so widely from that type, is usually capable of transmitting its extraordinary characters indefinitely by a-sexual, and not infrequently also by sexual, methods. So that, altogether, it seems impossible to suppose that in millions and millions of sister-buds, which through years and years exhibit no variation, a highly peculiar admixture of germ-plasm (which was originally present in the parent-seed) should have been latent; that it should then suddenly become so patent in a single bud, after which it never occurs in any other bud, save in the progeny of the sporting one.

On the whole, then, while it thus seems impossible to attribute all cases of bud-variation to mixtures of germ-plasms in sexual propagation, the theory of germ-plasm is unable to entertain any other explanation, on pain of surrendering its postulate touching the unalterable stability of germ-plasm, on which the Weismannian theory of evolution is founded.

So much for Weismann's evidence touching the extreme, or virtually everlasting, stability of germ-plasm. We have seen that this evidence is not merely of a very poor character *per se*, or on antecedent grounds; but that it is directly negatived as evidence by the a-sexual origin of species in the plants alluded to by Professor Vines; by certain facts which prove so high a degree of instability on the part of this hypothetical substance, that in some cases it admits of being very considerably modified in the course of only two or three generations by exposure to changed conditions of life; while in other cases it may "sport," so as to produce "hereditary individual variations," which are much more pronounced than any of those that ordinarily result from a blending of hereditary qualities in an act of sexual union.

It will be well to conclude our examination of Weismann's system by stating exactly the effect produced on his theory of evolution by the foregoing disproof of its fundamental postulate—the absolute stability of germ-plasm.

Clearly, in the first place, if germ-plasm has not been absolutely stable "since the first origin of sexual propagation," the hereditary characters of germ-plasm may have been modified any number of times, and in always accumulating degrees. It matters not whether the modifications have been due mainly to external or to internal causes. It is enough to have shown that modifications occur. For, it will be remembered, the doctrine of the absolute stability of germ-plasm is, that inasmuch as the "molecular" structure of germ-plasm cannot be affected either from without or from within, the only source of "hereditary individual variations" is to be found in admixtures of germ-plasms taking place in sexual fertilization. Slight "molecular" differences having been originally impressed upon different masses of germ-plasm when these were severally derived from their unicellular sources, so unalterable has been the stability of germ-plasm ever since, that these slight "molecular" differences have never been in any degree effaced; and although in sexual unions they have for untold ages been obliged to mix in ever-varying proportions, they still continue—and ever must continue—to assert themselves in each ontogeny. Therefore, as Weismann himself formulates this astonishing doctrine,—"The origin of hereditary individual variations cannot indeed be found in the higher organisms, the Metazoa and Metaphyta; but is to be sought for in the lowest—the unicellular organisms." Or again,—"The formation of new species, which among the lower Protozoa could be achieved without amphigony, could only be attained by means of this process in the Metazoa and Metaphyta. It was only in this way that hereditary individual differences could arise and persist[31]."

Now this doctrine is the most distinctive, as it is the most original feature in Weismann's system of theories. That it is of interest as an example of boldly carrying the premises of a theory to their logical termination, no one will deny. But as little can it be denied that the very stringency of this logical process brings the theory itself into collision with such facts as those which have now been stated, and which, as far as I can see, are destructive of the theory—or, at any rate, of all that side of the theory which depends on the doctrine of absolute stability.

Take, for instance, the sequent doctrine that natural selection is inoperative among the unicellular organisms. Here, indeed, we have another of those doctrines which are so improbable on merely antecedent grounds, that their presence might well be deemed a source of irremediable weakness to the whole theory of evolution of which they form integral, or logically essential, parts. For seeing that the rate of increase in most of the unicellular organisms is quite as high as—and in most cases very much higher than—the rate that obtains in any of the multicellular, it becomes on merely antecedent grounds incredible that the struggle for existence should here *not* lead to any survival of the fittest. When, for instance, we learn from Maupas that a single Stylonichia is potentially capable of yielding a billion descendants within a week, we should need some extraordinarily good evidence to make us believe that as regards this organism natural selection is inoperative. But the point at present is that, quite apart from all general and *a priori* considerations of this kind, Weismann's doctrine that unicellular organisms cannot be influenced by natural selection must be abandoned. For this doctrine followed deductively from the premiss that in the multicellular organisms congenital variations can only be due to admixtures of germ-plasms in acts of sexual fertilization; so that, in the absence of such admixtures, there could be no material for natural selection to work upon. But now we have found that this premiss must be given up; and, therefore, the deduction with respect to the unicellular organisms falls to the ground. Although it is true that the unicellular organisms propagate by fission, and although we grant, for the sake of argument, that they never propagate by way of sexual unions—even so this can no longer be taken to argue that none of their innumerable species owe their origin to natural selection. And, although it is probably true that the sexual methods of propagation constitute one source of hereditary individual variation among the multicellular organisms, there is no vestige of any independent reason for supposing that this is the *only* source of such variation; while the sundry facts which have now been given amount to nothing short of a demonstration to the contrary[32].

Lastly, and as regards the multicellular organisms, it is evident that Weismann's essay *On the Significance of Sexual Reproduction in the Theory of Natural Selection* must be cancelled. For, apart from the contradictory manner in which this matter has been stated (pp. 70, 93, notes), and apart also from the consideration that other and quite as probable reasons have been suggested for the origin of sexual reproduction, there is the fact that Weismann's theory is no longer tenable after the above destruction of its logical postulate in the absolute stability of germ-plasm. For, in the absence of this postulate, there is no basis for the theory that admixtures of germ-plasms in sexual reproduction furnish the sole means whereby heritable variations can be supplied for the working of natural selection.

Summary.

THE theory of germ-plasm is not only a theory of heredity: it is also, and more distinctively, a theory of evolution. As a theory of heredity it is grounded on its author's fundamental postulate—the continuity of germ-plasm; and, further, on a fact well recognized by all other theories of heredity, which he expresses by the term stability of germ-plasm. But as a theory of evolution it requires two additional postulates for its support—viz., that germ-plasm has been *perpetually* continuous "since the first origin of life," and *absolutely* stable "since the first origin of sexual reproduction." It is clear that these two additional postulates are not needed for his theory of heredity, but only for his additional theory of evolution. There have been other theories of heredity, prior to this one, which, like it, have been founded on the postulate of "continuity" (in Weismann's sense) of the substance of heredity; but it has not been needful for any of these theories to postulate further that this substance has been *always* thus isolated, or even that it is now *invariably* so. For even though the isolation be frequently invaded by influences of body-changes on the congenital characters of this substance, it does not follow that the body-changes must be transmitted to offspring exactly as they occurred in parents. They may produce in offspring what we have agreed to call "specialized" hereditary changes, even if they never produce "representative" hereditary changes,—i.e., the transmission of acquired characters. But it is essential to Weismann's theory of *evolution* that body-changes should not exercise a modifying influence of *any* kind on the ancestral endowments of this substance; hence, for the purposes of this further theory he has to assume that germ-plasm presents, not only *continuity*, but continuity *unbroken since the first origin of life*.

Similarly as regards his postulate of the stability of germ-plasm as *absolute*. It is enough for all the requirements of his theory of heredity, that the substance in question should present the high degree of stability which the facts of atavism, persistence of vestigial organs, &c., prove it to possess. But for his further theory of evolution it is necessary to make this further postulate of the stability of germ-plasm *as undisturbed since the first origin of sexual propagation*: otherwise there would be no logical foundation for any of the distinctive doctrines which go to constitute that theory.

Thus much understood, we proceeded to examine the theory of germ-plasm in each of its departments separately—i.e., first as a theory of heredity, and next as a theory of evolution. And we begun by comparing it as a theory of heredity with the preceding theories of Darwin and Galton. In the result we found that germ-plasm resembles gemmules in all the following respects. It is particulate; constitutes the material basis of heredity; is mainly lodged in highly specialized cells; is nevertheless also distributed throughout the general cellular tissues, where it is concerned in all processes of regeneration, repair, and a-sexual reproduction; presents an enormously complex structure, in that every constituent part of a potentially future organism is represented in a fertilized ovum by corresponding particles; is everywhere capable of virtually unlimited multiplication, without ever losing its hereditary endowments; is often capable of carrying these endowments in a dormant state through a long series of generations, until at last they reappear again in what we recognize as reversions. Such being the points of resemblance, the only points of difference may be summed up in the two words—continuity, and stability. For, as regards continuity, while Darwin's theory supposes the substance of heredity to be more or less formed anew in each generation by the body-tissues of that generation, Weismann's theory regards this substance as owing nothing to the body-tissues, further than lodgement and nutrition. Therefore, while the theory of gemmules can freely entertain the doctrines of Lamarck, the theory of germ-plasm excludes them as physiologically impossible, in all cases where sexual reproduction is concerned. Again, as regards stability, while Darwin's theory simply accepts the fact of such a degree of stability appertaining to the substance of heredity as the phenomena of atavism, &c. prove, Weismann's theory postulates the stability of this substance as absolute. But, as we have now so often seen, he does so in order to provide a hypothetical basis for his further theory of evolution. In as far as his theory of heredity is concerned, there is no reason why it should differ from Darwin's in this respect.

Again, comparing Weismann's theory of heredity with that of Galton, we found that germ-plasm resembles stirp in all the points wherein we have just seen that it resembles germ-plasm. Or, otherwise stated, all three theories are thus far coincident. But germ-plasm resembles stirp much more closely than it does gemmules, seeing that the theory of stirp is founded on the postulate of "continuity" in exactly the same manner as is the theory of germ-plasm. In point of fact, the only difference between these two theories consists in the two further postulates presented by the latter—viz., that the "continuity" in question has been unbroken since the origin of life, while the "stability" in question has been uninterrupted since the origin of sexual propagation. But seeing that both these additional postulates have reference to Weismann's theory of evolution, we may say that his theory of heredity is, as regards all essential points, indistinguishable from that of Galton.

The truly scientific attitude of mind with regard to the problem of heredity is to say, as Galton says, "that we might almost reserve our belief that the structural [i.e., somatic] cells can react on the sexual elements at all, and we may be confident that at most they do so in a very faint degree; in other words, that acquired modifications are barely, if at all, *inherited*, in the correct sense of that word." But for Weismann's further theory of evolution, it is necessary to postulate the two additional doctrines in question; and it makes a literally immeasurable difference to the theory of evolution whether or not we entertain these two additional postulates. For no matter how faintly or how fitfully the substance of heredity may be modified by somatic tissues, by external conditions of life, or even by so-called spontaneous changes on the part of this substance itself, numberless causes of congenital variation are thus admitted, while even the Lamarckian principles are hypothetically allowed some degree of play. And although this is a lower degree than Darwin supposed, their influence in determining the course of organic evolution may still have been enormous; seeing that their action in any degree must always have been *directive* on the one hand, and *cumulative* on the other.

Having thus pointed out the great distinction between the theories of stirp and of germ-plasm, it became needful to note that Weismann himself is not consistent in observing it. On the contrary, in some passages he apparently expresses himself as willing to resign both his distinctive postulates—continuity as *perpetual*, and stability as *absolute*. But it is evident that such passages must be ignored by his critics, because, although as far as his theory of heredity is concerned they betoken an approach to the less speculative views of Galton, any such approach is proportionally destructive of his theory of evolution. It must not be supposed that I am taking an ungenerous advantage of these occasionally fundamental concessions. On the contrary, one cannot but admire the candour which they display. But, as I have said, it is necessary for us to ignore them, if only in order to examine the Weismannian theory of germ-plasm as a distinctive theory at all. And more than this. Seeing that his theory of heredity differs from Galton's chiefly in being further an elaborate theory of evolution (founded on the two additional postulates in question), my main object has been to show the enfeeblement of the former which Weismann has caused by his addition of the latter. If he were to express his willingness to abandon his theory of evolution for the sake of strengthening his theory of heredity by identifying its main features with those of Galton's, personally I should have no criticism to pass. Indeed, I was myself one of the first evolutionists who called in question the Lamarckian factors; and ever since the publication of Galton's theory of heredity at about the same time, I have felt that in regard to its main principles—or those in which it agrees with Weismann's—it is probably the true one. But I can nowhere find that Weismann is thus prepared to surrender his theory of evolution. Occasionally he plays fast and loose with the two additional postulates on which this theory is founded; but he does so without appearing to perceive the speculative impossibility of any longer sustaining his temple of evolution if he were to remove its pillars of germ-plasm.

Ignoring, then, these inconsistencies, we proceeded to examine separately, and on their own respective merits, the two distinctive postulates of the theory of germ-plasm— *perpetual* continuity since the first origin of life, and *absolute* stability since the first origin of sexual propagation.

It does not appear to me that very much has to be said, either for or against the former postulate, on merely antecedent grounds, or grounds of general reasoning. Therefore I relegated to an Appendix my examination of what Weismann has argued on these grounds, while in the text I considered only what he has advanced as evidence *a posteriori*. Here, as we saw, he has developed three distinct lines of verification—viz. (A) the migration of germ-cells in some of the *Hydromedusae*,(B) the early separation of germ-cells in the ontogeny of certain Invertebrata, and (C) the alleged invariability of organisms which are produced parthenogenetically. But we have seen, with respect to (A), that the specialized character of germinal cells is a fact which every theory of heredity must more or less recognize; and, therefore, that the migration of these cells, wherever it may be found to occur, does not lend any peculiar countenance to Weismann's theory. There may be many reasons for such migration other than the one which this theory assigns; while the reason which it does assign is rendered improbable by the consideration that in the *Hydromedusae* the material of heredity is already and richly diffused throughout the general tissues. (B) and (C) are both contrary to fact; and, therefore, in whatever measure they would have corroborated the theory had they proved to be true, in that measure must they be held to discountenance the theory now that they have been shown to be false.

It appears, then, that there is no evidence in support of the postulate of the *perpetual* continuity of germ-plasm. There is nothing to show the necessary non-inheritance of acquired characters. The only evidence which one can recognize as good, is that which makes equally in favour of the theory of stirp—or rather, of the well-known fact that congenital characters are at any rate much *more* heritable than are acquired: which, it is needless to repeat, is a widely different thing from proving—or even rendering probable—the *absolute* restriction of germ-plasm to a separate "sphere" of its own "since the origin of life."

But now, although there is no evidence in support of this postulate, there is no small amount of evidence against it. For this evidence goes to indicate that no small amount of reciprocal action habitually takes place between body-tissues and germinal elements: indeed it seems almost to prove that the orbits of germ-plasm and somato-plasm are not mutually exclusive, but touch and cut each other to a considerable extent. The evidence in question, it will be remembered, is derived from the effects of puberty, senility, castration, &c.; the occasional effect of pollenization on the somatic tissues of plants; the influence which a stock occasionally exercises upon a scion, or *vice versa*, which proves the possibility of a transmission of hereditary characters by a mere grafting together of somatic tissues; the direct evidence given by De Vries that in certain Algae constituents of cellular tissue pass immediately from the maternal ovum to the daughter organism; and the evidence, both direct and indirect, which remains to be given on a larger scale in my subsequent volume, where we shall have to challenge the validity of Weismann's fundamental postulate touching the non-occurrence of Lamarckian factors in any of the multicellular organisms.

It must here again be noticed that in those passages where he concedes the possibly "occasional" transmission of acquired characters Weismann is annihilating his own theory, root and branch. Thus, for example, in allusion to De Vries' observation just mentioned, he says that we cannot exclude the possibility of "changes being induced by external conditions in the organism as a whole, and then communicated to the germ-cells after the manner indicated in Darwin's hypothesis of pangenesis." But it is obvious that the theory of germ-plasm *must* "exclude the possibility of such a transmission occasionally occurring"; for the very essence of that theory consists in its postulating a difference between germ-plasm and the general body-substance *in kind*, such that there never *can* be any "communication" from the one to the other "after the manner indicated by Darwin's hypothesis of pangenesis." Any prevarication over this point amounts simply to abandoning the theory of germ-plasm altogether, and opening up a totally distinct issue—namely, the *relative importance* of natural selection and the Lamarckian factors in the process of organic evolution. It may be perfectly true—and I myself believe it is perfectly true—that Darwin attributed too large a measure of importance to the Lamarckian factors; but whether or not he did so is quite a different question from that which obtains between his theory of pangenesis and Weismann's theory of germ-plasm. The former question is whether we are to "*modify*" the theory of pangenesis, so as to constitute it the theory of stirp; the latter question is whether we are to "*abolish*" the theory of pangenesis, in favour of its logical antithesis, the theory of germ-plasm. And this question remains to be dealt with in my next volume.

Coming then, lastly, to the companion postulate of germ-plasm as absolutely stable since the first origin of sexual propagation, we had to observe that, unlike the one we have just been considering, there is an immensely strong presumption against it on merely antecedent grounds. That the most complex substance in nature should likewise be the most stable substance with regard to complexity of "molecular structure"; that the greater its complexity becomes the greater becomes its stability, so that while in the comparatively simple unicellular organisms it is eminently susceptible of modification by external conditions, it entirely ceases to be thus susceptible when it becomes evolved into the incomparably more complex and immensely more varied structures which form the bases of heredity in the multicellular organisms—where, also, it must come into ever more and more intricate as well as more and more diverse relations with the external world;—all this is, I repeat, well nigh incredible. At any rate, speaking for myself, I should require some enormous weight of evidence to balance so enormous an antecedent improbability, or before I could regard such a doctrine as meriting any serious attention.

What, then, is the evidence that has been adduced? We have found that this evidence is *nil*. On the other hand, we have found that the evidence against the doctrine is abundantly sufficient to annihilate the doctrine—and this quite apart from all the antecedent considerations just alluded to. For not only have we the sundry facts of bud-variation, a-sexual origin of species, &c., which contradict the doctrine; but we have also the results of direct experiment, which prove that the alleged stability of germ-plasm may be conspicuously upset by slight changes in the external conditions of life. So that both from within and from without the stability which is alleged in theory admits of being overturned by facts.

And here, in order to avoid all possible confusion, I must ask it once more to be noted that there is not, and never has been, any question touching the *high degree* of stability which is exhibited by whatever substance it is that constitutes the material basis of heredity. But this is a widely different thing from supposing the stability *absolute*, so that it can never have been affected in any degree since the first origin of multicellular organisms, or in any of the millions of species into which these organisms have ramified. And the fact that in some cases we are actually able to observe a change of congenital characters as resulting from some "spontaneous" change in the hereditary material itself (as in bud-variation), or from some change in the external conditions of life (as in Hoffmann's experiments)—this fact is more than is required in order finally to overthrow the intrinsically untenable doctrine which is in question.

Now, with the collapse of this doctrine there collapses also the important chain of deductions therefrom, which together constitute Weismann's new theory of evolution. In particular, that natural selection is the exclusive means of modification among all the Metazoa and Metaphyta, while it is as exclusively ruled out with respect to all the Protozoa and Protophyta; that individual variations among the former can only be determined by sexual unions, while among the latter they can only be determined by the direct action of the environment; that the origin of congenital variability in all the Metazoa and Metaphyta is to be sought, and can only be found, in variations which occurred millions of years ago in the Protozoa and Protophyta; that the "significance of sexual propagation" is to be found in the view, that by this means alone can congenital variations have been ever since produced; &c., &c.

Upon the whole then, it appears to me that both the fundamental postulates of the theory of germ-plasm are unsound. That the substance of heredity is largely continuous and highly stable I see many and cogent reasons for believing. But that this substance has been uninterruptedly continuous since the origin of life, and absolutely stable since the origin of sexual propagation, I see even more and better reasons for disbelieving. And inasmuch as these two latter, or distinctive, postulates are not needed for Weismann's theory of heredity, while they are both essential to his theory of evolution, I cannot but regret that he should thus have crippled the former by burdening it with the latter. Hence my object throughout has been to display, as sharply as possible, the contrast that is presented between the brass and the clay in the colossal figure which Weismann has constructed. Hence, also, my emphatic dissent from his theory of evolution does not prevent me from sincerely appreciating the great value which attaches to his theory of heredity. And although I have not hesitated to say that this theory is, in my opinion, incomplete; that it presents not a few manifest inconsistencies, and even logical contradictions; that the facts on which it is founded have always been facts of general knowledge; that in all its main features it was present to the mind of Darwin, and distinctly formulated by Galton; that in so far as it has been constituted the basis of a more general theory of organic evolution, it has clearly proved a failure:—such considerations in no wise diminish my cordial recognition of the services which its distinguished author has rendered to science by his speculations upon these topics. For not only has he been successful in drawing renewed and much more general attention to the important questions touching the transmissibility of acquired characters, the causes of variation, and so on; but even those parts of his system which have proved untenable are not without such value as temporary scaffoldings present in relation to permanent buildings. Therefore, if I have appeared to play the *rôle* of a hostile critic, this has only been an expression of my desire to separate what seems to me the grain of good science from the chaff of bad speculation. And the candour which Professor Weismann has always displayed towards criticism of this character enables me to hope with assurance, that I have said nothing which he himself will regard as inconsistent with high admiration of his work as a naturalist, or of his originality as a philosopher.

CHAPTER V.

WEISMANNISM UP TO DATE (1893).

HITHERTO we have been considering Professor Weismann's system as it stood prior to the publication of his most recent works on *Amphimixis* and *The Germ-plasm*, in 1891 and 1893 respectively. These later and highly elaborate essays present considerable modifications of the system, as it stood when the foregoing criticism was written. But, for reasons already stated in the Preface, it appears to me desirable to leave that criticism as it was originally constructed, and to supply this further chapter for the purpose of dealing with the large alterations of, and important additions to, the theory of germ-plasm, which the maturer thought of its gifted author has led him to announce.

A few general remarks may be most conveniently made at the outset.

In the first place, these recent publications present the advantage over their predecessors of being systematic treatises, instead of more or less independent papers. On this account they present a logical sequence of thought, which renders the task of examination much less difficult than it was in the case of the first volume of the *Essays*.

In the second place, as a result of his more matured reflection, Professor Weismann has himself perceived a considerable number of the difficulties and objections which I have set forth in the preceding chapters. And not only has he thus anticipated many of my criticisms; but, as a result of doing so, he has changed not a few of the most important parts of his previous system, with the result of greatly improving it.

But, in the third place, notwithstanding that his remarkable power of speculative thinking is everywhere united with adequate knowledge in the sundry branches of biological science with which it deals, I confess to a serious doubt whether it has not been permitted to enjoy an undue amount of liberty. If only they can be laced together by a thread of logical connexion, hypotheses are added to hypotheses in such profusion as we are acquainted with in the works of metaphysicians, but which has rarely been approached in those of naturalists. The whole mechanism of heredity has been now planned out in such minuteness of detail and assurance of accuracy, that in reading the account one is reminded of that which is given by Dante of the topography of Inferno. For not only is the "sphere" of germ-plasm now composed of nine circles (molecules, biophores, determinants, ids, idants, idio-plasm, somatic-idioplasm, morpho-plasm, apical-plasm), but in most of these regions our guide is able to show us such strange and interesting phenomena, that we return to the fields of science with a sense of having been indeed in some other world. Or, to change the metaphor, if it be the case that "a true scientific judgement consists in giving a free rein to speculation with one hand, while holding ready the break of verification with the other," I think it must be admitted that, in as far as he has erred, Professor Weismann has done so by driving a chariot which is unprovided with any break at all.

Hence, fourthly, it is needless to follow, even in epitome, the innumerable windings of these never-ending speculations. For, on the one hand, it would be impossible to do so without adding an unduly extended chapter to our already tediously prolonged consideration of Weismann's views; while, on the other hand, we should have to deal merely with matters of comparative detail. The additions which have been made to his theory by his most recent publications are chiefly concerned with the matter just alluded to—viz., a minute elaboration of the hypothetical mechanism of heredity, in accordance with the general theory of germ-plasm. Without question this elaboration is everywhere thoughtful, and often highly ingenious; but until the general theory in question shall have been satisfactorily grounded, it seems premature to supply so immense a design of purely deductive construction. Beautiful though it may be in its imposing elevation, this drawing of "the architecture of germ-plasm" must be regarded as a work of artistic imagination rather than as one of scientific generalization. From the latter point of view it is at most a temple *in posse*, and even if it is ever to be realized *in esse*, we cannot allow the actual building to begin until we are much more sure than anybody is at present entitled to be touching the foundations on which it is proposed to rear so great an edifice.

Again, and fifthly, even if Weismann should ever be able to satisfy us upon this matter, or fully to demonstrate his basal proposition touching the perpetual continuity of germ-plasm, there would still be a far cry between accepting this sufficiently simple proposition and supposing that there is any adequate reason for entertaining so complex a scheme of the structure of germ-plasm. No doubt Weismann himself would be quite ready to admit, that from his basal proposition of the continuity of germ-plasm it is logically possible to construct many other designs of the architecture of germ-plasm, besides the one which he has so beautifully drawn. And although most of such alternative designs would doubtless embody some one or other of the features which are presented by his own, no one could say which features common to any two of the designs represent the facts. For in the case of all alike there would be a necessary absence of verification: the architects would all and equally have to acknowledge that their imposing pictures of "the palace of truth" were but imaginary. Such, in my opinion, has been the case with all theories of the ultimate mechanism of heredity hitherto published; but the difference between them and Weismann's theory in this respect is, that while most of the others have not gone into speculative details further than was necessary as a means of substantiating their basal postulates, Weismann's, as now developed in *The Germ-plasm*, is mainly concerned with such speculative details as an end, or object, *per se*.

But, it may be replied, by thus constructing an ideal mechanism of heredity Weismann is greatly strengthening his fundamental postulate of the continuity of germ-plasm, because he shows how all the main facts of heredity, and allied phenomena, admit of being explained if once the postulate be accepted. If this were urged, however, I should have two remarks to offer. The first is that Weismann, in constructing his ideal mechanism, has gone very much further in the way of elaboration than can possibly be required for this purpose. So much further, indeed, that his purpose has evidently been the constructing of his ideal mechanism, as I have just said, for its own sake, and not for the sake of substantiating its basal proposition by showing how well the latter can be made to work in explaining the phenomena of heredity, &c. Moreover—and this is my second remark—however well the basal proposition may be made to work in this respect, we must not be deceived into supposing that such a fact is equivalent to a substantiation of the proposition. This proposition—the continuity of germ-plasm—is the inverse of that which constitutes the basis of the theory of pangenesis. For while the latter assumes that in the last resort it is always somatic tissues which produce the substance of heredity, the former simply inverts the terms of this assumption, and holds that it is always the substance of heredity which produces the somatic tissues. Now, in all cases where one theory consists in thus simply inverting the terms of another, it will be found that the facts which they both seek to explain lend themselves equally to explanation by either, up to some certain and usually distant point, where a crucial test becomes possible. Take, as an example, the geocentric and heliocentric theories of the solar system. Here the question was whether the earth moved round the sun, or *vice versa*; and so many of the facts of observation lent themselves equally well to either interpretation, that it was very many centuries before the crucial tests were forthcoming. So, in the present instance, the question is as to whether the carriers of heredity move from body-cells to germ-cells, or *vice versa*; and it is because the theory which sustains the latter view has merely to invert the terms of the one which takes the former, that so many of the facts of observation lend themselves equally well to both—as we have seen in chapter III (pp. 56-59).

Lastly, yet another reason for not considering in any detail Professor Weismann's intricate speculations on the ultimate mechanism of heredity is, that by so doing I should have found it impossible to avoid obscuring the main issues. For even Professor Weismann himself, by the extreme care which he has taken in fully presenting his scheme of this ultimate mechanism, has not found it practicable to keep distinctly before our view the relative insignificance of such details, as compared with the fundamental importance of his original postulates. Hence, I have deemed it best in the present chapter to restrict our attention to the changes which he has recently made in these the foundations of his entire system.

For these reasons, then, I will mention only those main features in the "architecture of germ-plasm" which it is necessary to understand for the purposes of the following criticism touching the general theory of germ-plasm in the most recent phase of its evolution.

To begin with, Weismann has now seen the desirability of ceasing to designate the ultimate "carriers of heredity" by the term "molecules." Indeed, in these later volumes he has fully anticipated my remarks touching the use of this term in his previous "Essays[33]." The result of his more mature reflection may be presented in epitome thus.

A number of "molecules," in the proper or chemical sense of the word, go to form a "biophore," which is the ultimate unit of living substance.

A number of " biophores" go to form a "determinant," which is a special element in the germ-plasm, capable of directing the ontogeny of such and such a group of cells as is independently variable from the germ onwards.

A number of "determinants" go to form an "id," which is the same hypothetical body as Weismann has hitherto designated by the term "ancestral germ-plasm." That is to say, it is a group of determinants indissolubly united in phylogeny, and therefore transmitted by heredity as one complex whole. Ids are, perhaps, microscopically visible; and, if so, they probably correspond to the small granules (microsomata), which are familiar to the histologist in the structure of chromosomes.

A number of "ids" go to form an "idant," which is a chromosome, or chromatin fibre[34].

In my opinion the most important advance which Weismann has made in his theory by means of this scheme has reference to the third of these divisions—the determinant. It is a matter of observation that every cell of a multicellular organism does not vary independently: it appears to be always the case that in the phenomena of variation a smaller or a larger *group* of cells is concerned. Now there must be something that determines the similar and simultaneous variation of such a whole group of cells; and, in all cases where such a variation is congenital, it is certain that this something must be contained in the substance of heredity. So far, I think, we must all agree, whether or not we regard this substance as "germ-plasm." In other words, whether we regard the carriers of heredity as proceeding centrifugally (germ-plasm) or centripetally (gemmules), it seems to me that we ought to accept Weismann's doctrine of determinants. Indeed, pathologists have already furnished a foreshadowing of such a doctrine in regard to the phenomena presented by certain diseases, such as cancer; but it is an important step to have extended the idea from pathology to biology in general—and, at the same time, to have given it a more definite shape than it has hitherto presented. In Weismann's hands it serves to render more conceivable—if not also more intelligible—that process of marshalling cell-formations, which, be our theories what they may, is assuredly the most distinctive and remarkable fact of ontogenetic organization.

Again, as regards the id, I do not see how any one can attentively read Professor Weismann's discussion without acknowledging that, if we once accept his doctrine of determinants, his sequent doctrine of ids becomes a logical necessity.

On the other hand, however, I do not see that such is the case with respect to idants; and still less do I see any reason for identifying the latter with chromosomes—even assuming that chromosomes are the visible repositories of the carriers of heredity[35].

Referring the reader to Weismann's own exposition for a full account of these and many other additions to his general theory of germ-plasm, I will at once proceed to consider the alterations or emendations of that theory which have been published in his last two volumes, and which, as we shall find, have in large measure anticipated some of the most important points in the foregoing criticism. Therefore in the following criticism I will consider *seriatim* what he has now said touching all these points, and conclude by offering some general remarks on the resulting position of his general system of theories up to the present date.

Pursuing the same method of criticism as that adopted in the preceding chapters, we will first consider the further modifications of Weismann's theory of heredity, and next those of his theory of organic evolution.

Weismann's theory of Heredity (1893).

First of all, Weismann has now profoundly modified his theory of polar bodies. For, owing to certain more recent researches of Professor O. Hertwig, he very candidly allows:—"My previous interpretation of the first polar body as the removal of ovogenetic nucleo-plasm from the egg must fall to the ground: about this there is no possible doubt[36]."

He now regards both polar bodies as concerned in the same function of removing superfluous germ-plasm. Therefore one-half of his previous theory is abandoned: "the ovogenetic idio-plasm" is now supposed to be simply absorbed in the course of ontogeny, as I had suggested in one of the preceding chapters (pp. 42-46). The consequence is that he has now nothing to oppose to the view which is likewise there suggested (pp. 43-44)—viz., that his whole theory of polar bodies is rendered needless and improbable by the fact that the very mode in which ova are produced renders ample provision for the removal of any amount of superfluous germ-plasm which the theory of germ-plasm may require.

It is needless to say, after what has already been said in the pages just referred to, that in my opinion Professor Weismann has improved his main system of theories by dropping this part of his subordinate and, for the most part, separate theory of polar bodies. I only wish he could have seen his way to dropping the whole.

Again, he has now fully considered the phenomena of repair, regeneration, reproduction from somatic tissues, budding, and graft-hybridization.

Touching the four former he takes the view which I have supposed that he would (p. 53). As regards the latter, he fully accepts the fact of an occasional transmission of characters from one species or variety of plant to another by mere grafting[37]. But, although the explanation which he gives of this fact may pass muster so far as the only case which he deals with in detail is concerned, I do not see how it can do so to many others. For the case which he considers is that of *Cystisus adami*, where a bud of one species of Laburnum having been inserted in the wood of another produced a shoot which presented intermediate characters; and these have ever since been propagated by cuttings. Weismann's interpretation of the facts here is, "that they were due to an abnormal kind of amphimixis, so that the idants of both species were combined in the apical cell of the first shoot[38]." Now, although this explanation may well apply to a case of graft-hybridization by means of buds, it obviously cannot do so to any case where hybridization is produced by the grafting of woody tissues. For here there is no "apical cell" in the question; and therefore the difficulties which I have adduced on page 82 remain. Possibly Weismann may dispute the fact of hybridization in any of these cases; but, as he has not expressly done so, I will not go into the question of evidence[39].

One important addition to this side of Weismann's system has been made in order to meet the class of difficulties which are presented by the apparent inheritance of certain climatic variations, as already mentioned on pp. 67-8. For example, his own butterflies seemed to render definite proof of somatogenetic variations caused by changed conditions of life being transmitted to progeny. Therefore, it will be remembered, Weismann candidly admitted, "even now I cannot explain the facts otherwise than by supposing a passive acquisition of characters produced by the direct influence of climate"—i.e., an exactly *representative* copying in progeny of characters acquired by parents. I have already quoted these words in order to show their logical inadmissibility as used by Weismann. He cannot be allowed thus to entertain the Lamarckian factors and at the same time to maintain his theory of germ-plasm, which excludes them as physiologically impossible. Doubtless he was himself aware of this, for he immediately added that "new experiments will be necessary to afford the *true* explanation[40]."

The explanation, however, which he now gives is not based on any new experiments, but on a new suggestion to the effect that all such seemingly conclusive instances of the inheritance of acquired characters are, in truth, illusory. This suggestion is that "Many climatic variations may be due wholly or in part to the simultaneous variation of corresponding determinants in some parts of the soma, and in the germ-plasm of the reproductive cells.[41]" For example, if, as Weismann now supposes, determinants of the same kinds occur in the somatic tissues as well as in the germ-cells, when a particular spot occurs on a butterfly's wing, it has been due to a particular kind of determinant which in the course of ontogeny was transmitted from the germ-cell for the express purpose of controlling the size and colour of the spot. But a residue of precisely similar determinants was reserved in the germ-cell (germ-plasm), for the purpose of determining a precisely similar spot in the next generation. Hence, if a rise of temperature, or any other external change, is capable of so acting on the determinant in the soma as to cause it to impart an abnormal colour to the spot when formed, a similar change is likely to be simultaneously effected in the corresponding determinants which are lying dormant in the germ-plasm. Therefore, when the latter become active in the ontogeny of the next generation, they will produce spots presenting the same variations as those of the preceding generation. Obviously, however, there would not be here any transmission of acquired characters. The change would be "specialized," but not "representative."

No doubt we have here a sufficiently ingenious method of circumventing an awkward class of facts. But I should like to make two observations with regard to it.

In the first place, the suggestion is highly speculative, and has been advanced solely for the sake of saving the theory of germ-plasm. There are no facts adduced in its favour, and it could scarcely be entertained as in the least degree probable by any one who has not already accepted the theory in question. Hence, unless we are to embark on a course of circular reasoning, we must refuse to accept the explanation of hereditary climatic variation now offered, until it shall have been fully corroborated by the experimental enquiry to which Weismann says he is now submitting it.

My second observation is, that the suggestion is not new; but appears to have been derived from Professor Weismann's recent study of Mr. Galton's *Theory of Heredity*. At all events, the suggestion is there presented with sufficient lucidity, thus:—

> It is said that the structure of an animal changes when he is placed under changed conditions; that his offspring inherit some of his change; and that they vary still further on their own account, in the same direction, and so on through successive generations, until a notable change in the congenital characteristics of

the race has been effected. Hence, it is concluded that a change in the personal structure has reacted on the sexual elements. For my part, I object to so general a conclusion, for the following reasons. It is universally admitted that the primary agents in the processes of growth, nutrition, and reproduction are the same, and that a true theory of heredity must so regard them. In other words, they are all due to the development of some germinal matter, variously located. Consequently, when similar germinal matter is everywhere affected by the same conditions, we should expect that it would be everywhere affected in the same way. The particular kind of germ whence the hair sprang, that was induced to throw out a new variety in the cells nearest to the surface of the body under certain changed conditions of climate and food, might be expected to throw out a similar variety in the sexual elements at the same time. The changes in the germs would everywhere be collateral, although the moments when any of the changed germs happened to receive their development might be different[42].

This allusion to Mr. Galton's *Theory of Heredity* leads me to consider what Professor Weismann has said with regard to it in this latest publication, where, for the first time, he has dealt with it. In my opinion he has done but scant justice to the views of his predecessor, and therefore I will occupy some considerable space in seeking to justify this opinion.

As already stated, from the time that Mr. Galton published his theory I have felt that in its main contention it presents a probably true solution of the main problem of heredity—viz., to account for the contrast between congenital and acquired characters in respect of transmissibility. And this solution, as likewise already stated, was substantially identical with that which Professor Weismann published in the next decade. Indeed, the only important difference between these two theories of heredity is, that while Weismann's excludes on deductive grounds the physiological possibility of the inheritance of acquired characters, Galton's more judiciously leaves to be determined, by subsequent enquiry of the inductive kind, the question whether acquired characters are ever transmitted in faint degrees, or whether they are never transmitted at all. In addition to this important difference, however, there are certain others which seem to me of very little consequence, inasmuch as they have reference to speculations on the ultimate mechanism of heredity, or the intimate morphology and physiology of the carriers of heredity—speculations which it would be absurd to suppose can be other than purely conjectural. Therefore in my previous criticism I did not allude to these subordinate points of difference, but stated merely, in general terms, that Galton's view of the ultimate mechanism in question was such as to leave room for the possibility of the occasional transmission of acquired characters. And in this respect, it still seems to me, his theory has an advantage over that of Weismann. No doubt the latter is a much more elaborate and highly finished piece of work; but beauty of ideal construction is no guarantee of scientific truth—as we shall presently find exemplified in a striking manner with regard to Weismann's theory of evolution. And if his theory of heredity, in its final shape, is a much more precise, detailed, and logically coherent structure than any which has ever been framed in this department of biological thought, there is all the more reason to scan critically the fundamental postulate on which it rests. Hence I cannot help feeling that it will be time enough to consider minor differences between the two theories when the physiological possibility of the occasional transmission of acquired characters, as entertained by Galton's theory, shall have been ruled out as demonstrably opposed to fact.

Seeing, however, that Professor Weismann thinks otherwise, and appears to attach as much importance to differences concerning deductive *minutiae* as he does to those concerning fundamental principles, I will here contrast the two theories somewhat more in detail than heretofore, and with special reference to what he has now himself said touching their relationship.

It will be remembered that the primary or fundamental difference just alluded to is, that while the theory of germ-plasm postulates an *absolute* continuity, the theory of stirp postulates but a *partial* continuity, of the substance of heredity. Hence, according to Weismann's view, we must go back to the unicellular organisms for the origin of this substance in the multicellular; and we must regard use-inheritance as physiologically impossible. On the other hand, according to Galton's view, there is no necessity for us to do either of these things. The origin of stirp is to be found in the somatic tissues of the multicellular organisms themselves. Nevertheless, this theory differs greatly from pangenesis, in that the former supposes the origin of hereditary substance to be mainly given in the *phylogeny* of any group of multicellular organisms, while the latter supposes it to be given mainly in each *ontogeny*, Galton's theory is, that in each ontogeny only a small part of the stirp derived from parents is consumed in making the new organism— the larger part being handed over in trust for passing on to the next generation, in the same way as Weismann supposes to be the case with germ-plasm. Darwin's theory, on the other hand, does not entertain any such notion of "continuity" in the substance of heredity from germ-cell to germ-cell of parent and offspring; it supposes that in each successive generation the germ-cells are *wholly* supplied with their germinal material from somatic-cells of each individual organism. Or, adopting our previous terminology, the three theories may be ranked thus.

The particulate elements of heredity all proceed centripetally from somatic-cells to germ-cells (gemmules): the inheritance of acquired characters is therefore habitual.

These particulate elements proceed for the most part, though not exclusively, from germ-cells to somatic-cells (stirp): the inheritance of acquired characters is therefore but occasional.

The elements in question proceed exclusively in the centrifugal direction last mentioned (germ-plasm): the inheritance of acquired characters is therefore impossible[43].

Such being the fundamental points of difference between these three theories of heredity, we have now to consider more particularly those which obtain between Galton's and Weismann's.

The general doctrine of gemmules (i. e. somatic-cell-germs) is accepted by Galton; but instead of supposing, as Darwin supposed, that these minute bodies freely circulate through all the body tissues, so that some of them are absorbed from all the somatic-cells by the germ-cells, and there constitute the entire mass of hereditary material out of which the offspring will afterwards be formed, Galton supposes that gemmules circulate with comparative difficulty, and that only comparatively few of them gain access to the germ-cells in each generation. Hence, characters acquired in the individual lifetime are much less heritable than those which are called congenital. For congenital characters are due to the "continuity" of stirp through numberless generations in the phylogeny of the organism; hence such characters are represented by a vastly greater number of equivalent hereditary elements. Weismann, on the other hand, rejects the doctrine of gemmules *in toto*.

Again, according to Galton's view, "individual [congenital] variation depends upon two factors; the one is the variability of the germ[44] and of its progeny; the other is that of all kinds of external circumstances, in determining which out of many competing germs, of nearly equal suitability, shall be the one that becomes developed. The variability of germs under changed conditions, and that of their progeny, may be small, but it is indubitable; absolute uniformity being scarcely conceivable in the condition and growth, and, therefore, in the reproduction of any organism. The law of heredity goes no further than to say, that like *tends* to produce like; the tendency may be very strong, but it cannot be absolute[45]."

Here, of course, there is a wide difference between stirp and germ-plasm. For while Galton does not entertain amphimixis among the "factors" of congenital variation, Weismann, as we are now well aware, has hitherto regarded it as the sole cause of such variation. Nevertheless, as we shall presently find, Weismann has now greatly modified his views upon this point, and does entertain, in *The Germ-plasm*, both the "factors" mentioned by Galton. Hence, the difference between the two theories in question with regard to this matter is not nearly so wide as it was prior to the publication of Weismann's last work.

The next most important point of difference between the theories of stirp and germ-plasm has reference to the mechanism of ontogeny. According to Galton, this is simply a struggle between all the carriers of heredity composing the stirp of a fertilized ovum. It is not, however, a struggle for existence, but what may be called a struggle for development. In the fertilized ovum all the carriers of heredity are, to begin with, in a "latent" condition; but of this enormous multitude of "germs" or "gemmules," only a very small proportional number are destined to become "patent"—i. e., developed into the tissue-cells composing the new organism. The vast majority of the gemmules, or those which fail to be thus developed, go to constitute the stirp of the new organism when this has been formed by the development of the comparatively few successful gemmules. Thus much understood, the following quotation will be fully intelligible.

> My argument is this: Of the two groups of germs, the one consisting of those that succeed in becoming developed and in forming the bodily structure, and the other consisting of those that remain continually latent, the latent vastly preponderates in number. We should expect the latent germs to exercise a corresponding predominance in matters of heredity, unless it can be shown that, on the whole, the germ that is developed into a cell becomes thereby more fertile than if it had remained latent. But the evidence points the other way. It appears both that the period of fertility is shorter, and the fecundity even during that period is less in the germ that becomes developed into a cell, than they are in the germ that remains latent. Much less then would the entire bodily structure, which consists of a relatively small number of these comparatively sterile units, successfully compete in matters of heredity with the total effect of the much more numerous and more prolific units which are in a latent form[46].

Thus, Galton's theory of the mechanism of geny is a theory of struggle; and this constitutes a point of difference on which Weismann lays much stress in his latest work. For, as we know, Weismann regards the mechanism of ontogeny as characterized by a peaceful succession of "stages," which are "pre-determined from the germ onwards";

and in his latest work this idea of orderly sequence has been further elaborated in his doctrine of "determinants." In short, to adopt their own metaphors, while Galton tells us that the mechanism of ontogeny is like that of a political election, where rival candidates compete to "represent" the nation (stirp) in Parliament (individual organism); Weismann likens it to the mechanism of a well-drilled army, where ultimate carriers of heredity (privates) are banded together in companies, regiments, battalions, &c., under the command of corresponding officers (determinants).

Lastly, there is yet one further point of difference between stirp and germ-plasm, which is thus stated by Weismann:—

> Galton's idea is only conceivable on the presupposition of the occurrence of sexual reproduction, while the theory of the continuity of the germ-plasm is entirely independent of any assumption as to whether each primary constituent is present in the germ *singly* or in numbers. According to my idea, the active and the reserve germ-plasm contain precisely similar primary constituents, gemmules, or determinants; and on this the resemblance of a child to its parent depends. The theory of the continuity of the germ-plasm, as I understand it, is not based on the fact that each "gemmule" necessary for the construction of the soma is present many times only, so that a residue remains from which the germ-cells of the next generation may be formed: it is founded on the view of the existence of a special adaptation, which is inevitable in the case of multicellular organisms, and which consists in the germ-plasm of the fertilized egg-cell becoming doubled primarily, one of the resulting portions being reserved for the formation of germ-cells[47].

These being the main points of difference between the theories of stirp and of germ-plasm to which Professor Weismann has alluded, I will now proceed to consider them separately, in reverse order to that in which they have been here stated.

The point of difference last mentioned need not detain us long, because it seems to me one of very little importance. "Whether each primary constituent is present in the germ singly or in numbers" cannot greatly signify, so long as both theories agree that, sooner or later, they must be present plurally. Galton supposes them to be thus present from the first (i. e. in the unfertilized ovum), while Weismann supposes them to be so only as a result of their self-multiplication at a somewhat later stage (i. e. in the segmenting ovum, and onwards throughout the procreative life of the individual). Doubtless Weismann does not suppose that they ever become so numerous as Galton imagines; but the whole question is so highly speculative that I do not see how any useful purpose can be served by debating it. Nor do I see why Weismann should conclude that "Galton's idea is only conceivable on the presupposition of the occurrence of sexual reproduction." It is true that Galton has discussed exclusively the case of sexual reproduction; but I cannot perceive that any of his ideas are inapplicable to a-sexual.

Touching the question whether the phenomena of ontogeny had best be ascribed to a competition among a vast number of "germs," or to a strictly ordered evolution of a comparatively small number of "determinants," a considerable array of arguments might be adduced in support of either view. Thus, Galton might well maintain that his interpretation of the observable facts is most in accordance with the general analogies supplied by organic nature as a whole. The ancient aphorism of Heraclitus, "Struggle is the father, king, and lord of all things," has been in large measure justified by Darwin and his followers, at any rate within the range of biology. Not only have we the "struggle for existence" where "the origin of species" is concerned; but Roux has well argued, in his remarkable work on *Der Kampf der Theile im Organismus*, that the principle of "struggle" is concerned to an equally important extent as between all the constituent parts of the same individual. But if this is so—if every tissue-cell of the organism owes its maintenance to success in a general contest for nutriment, &c.,—do we not find at least a probability that it owes its origin as a visible cell to a similar success in a similarly general contest among the invisible elements from which tissue-cells are developed? Nay, does it not seem well nigh incredible that when this selection-principle is seen to be the governing cause of evolution everywhere else, it should cease to play any part at all just at the place where we are unable to see what is going on? As we are agreed that this "father of all things" is of prime importance in phylogeny—to say nothing of physiology, psychology, and sociology,—must we not deem it absurd to suppose that it is supplanted in ontogeny by the opposite principle of absolute peace?

On the other hand, Weismann adduces many forcible considerations *per contra*; so that, in the result, I deem it best to dispose of the question with two general remarks. The first is, that the rival views are not necessarily incompatible. Each may present one aspect of the truth. Weismann's doctrine of determinants may be—and, to the best of my judgement, must be—sound; but this does not hinder that Galton's doctrine of struggling "germs" may be so likewise. For, as we have already seen, these germs present the same compound character which belong to determinants; in fact I do not suppose that Galton would object to identifying them with determinants. On the other hand, I do not see why Weismann should object to supposing that similar determinants compete among themselves for ontogenetic development. Indeed, he has already argued, in his suggestive theory of "germ-tracts," that it is usually only one among a number of similar determinants which does succeed in achieving such development—or, as he expresses it, which "becomes active." But what is it that causes this activity? Surely it must be some superiority on the part of the active determinant over its passive companions. And, if so, it is the selection-principle that is here at work. In fact, he has himself laid no small stress on what he calls "the struggle of the determinants of the two parents in ontogeny," and has even supplied a long section on "the Struggle of the Ids in Ontogeny." Therefore I do not see why he should so emphatically dissent from Galton's view upon this matter as he does in his work on *The Germ-plasm*[48].

My second remark is a brief one—viz., that the whole question is of so very speculative a character, that I cannot see the smallest use in debating it.

The only remaining point of difference between strip and germ-plasm is the one referring to stability. Needless to say, Galton is at one with Weismann in recognizing a high degree of stability on the part of the substance of heredity; but the agreement extends only so far as is necessitated by the facts of atavism, &c. Indeed, he does not even mention—although he perhaps implies—what Weismann has called amphimixis as among the factors of individual congenital variation. Weismann, on the other hand, has hitherto regarded amphimixis as the sole cause of all such variations. But, as we shall presently find, in his recent work on *The Germ-plasm* he has now greatly modified his views upon this subject, and, in fully recognizing the "factors" of variability to which Galton alludes, has correspondingly lessened the difference between germ-plasm and stirp. But this is a point which can be better dealt with when we come to consider the important modifications which in this respect the theory of germ-plasm has undergone.

The only other matter which has to be mentioned in connexion with Weismann's theory of heredity is, that in *The Germ-plasm* he has for the first time given us his views upon the influence of a previous sire on the progeny of a subsequent one by the same dam. The phenomena in question, which I have already detailed in pp. 77-9, 110, he designates by the term "telegony." The analogous phenomena in plants he calls, following Focke, "xenia."

With regard to telegony, he adopts, almost precisely, the position which I surmised that he would. That is to say, he first disputes the alleged facts, and then argues that, even if they be facts, they admit of being explained on the theory of germ-plasm by supposing that some of the germ-plasm from the first sire penetrates the unripe ova which are afterwards fertilized by the second[49]. The only difference between his views and my own upon this matter is, therefore, as follows.

Supposing that the phenomena alleged ever occur in fact, I have said that the only way of explaining them would seem to be, "that the life of 'germ-plasm' is not conterminous with that of the spermatozoa which convey it, and hence that, if the carriers of heredity, after the disintegration of their containing spermatozoa, should ever penetrate an unripe ovum, the germ-plasm thus introduced might remain dormant in the ovum until the latter becomes mature, and is then fertilized by another sire. In this way it is conceivable that the hitherto dormant germ-plasm of the previous sire might exercise some influence on the ontogeny of the embryo[50]."

Now, this is substantially the position which Weismann takes up: only instead of supposing that it is the "carriers of heredity" of the first sire which gain access to the unripe ovum "after the disintegration of their containing spermatozoa," he supposes that it is one of the spermatozoa which does so before its disintegration has commenced. Of course there is here no difference in principle, but only a question touching the mode in which the access is presumably effected. But, as regards this question, I retain my original opinion. For, while I can see no theoretical difficulty in supposing that "the carriers of heredity," when set free by the disintegration of their containing spermatozoa, may reach the unripe ova while still embedded in the depths of the ovary, I do see a difficulty, amounting almost to a physiological impossibility, in supposing that a whole spermatozoon can perform such a feat. From all that we know about the powers and functions of spermatozoa in the vertebrata, it appears simply absurd to imagine that these bodies are able to penetrate the dense coating of an ovary, and then delve their way through the stroma. There is, indeed, a remarkable investigation which was published a year or two ago by Mr. Whitman[51] which appears to prove that in certain leeches the male injects his seminal fluid into any part of the body of the female, and that the spermatozoa then reach the ova by wandering about her general tissues until some of them happen to hit upon her ovary. But in this case the spermatozoa are specially adapted to perform such acts of penetration—being spear-like bodies provided with a sharp point. Hence, if Weismann should quote this instance, it would not tend to support his view, seeing that the spermatozoa of mammals do not exhibit any such specializations of structure; and therefore, before any one of them can effect fertilization, must wait for the ovum to mature, reach the surface of the ovary, and rupture its follicle.

But, as already observed, it does not signify, so far as we are here concerned with the matter, in what precise manner the telegonous influence may be supposed to be exercised—provided that it may be so *directly*, and not necessarily through first having to influence the whole material organism. Therefore I quite agree with Weismann that the facts—supposing them to be facts—are quite as explicable by the theory of germ-plasm as by that of pangenesis[52].

Again, with respect to xenia, Weismann writes:—

> As such eminent botanists as Focke, and more recently De Vries, have expressed much doubt with regard to these observations—or rather interpretations—we must wait until these cases have been critically re-investigated before attempting to account for them theoretically. The chief difficulty we should meet with in any such explanation would be due to the fact that we are here concerned with the influence of the *germ-plasm* of the sperm-cell on a tissue of another plant which only constitutes *a part* of this plant. It would thus be necessary to assume that all the determinants of this germ-plasm are not active, and that only those take effect which determine the nature of the fruit.

Now, it does not appear that De Vries has looked into the matter on his own account, as he merely refers to what Focke has said. And this amounts merely to showing the dubious character of some half-dozen cases which Focke gives as those which alone have fallen within his cognizance. Why he does not mention any of the numerous cases which are quoted by Darwin, I do not understand. Nor can I understand why he does not consider what seem to be the particularly conclusive facts given on p. 80,—i. e., where xenia appears to constitute "a needful preliminary to fertilization." But the whole matter is one for botanists to deal with, and if any doubt attaches to it, at least the grounds of such doubt should be fully stated. Still more, in my opinion, should the matter be freed from any such doubt. The question—if there be a question—is one of great interest from a merely physiological point of view, while in relation to the fundamental problems of heredity its importance is immense. Surely, then, any competent botanist who disputes the facts ought to test them by way of experiment.

But, be this as it may, I must call prominent attention to the following very remarkable words wherewith Weismann concludes the passage above quoted. For he there says, that even supposing there were no doubt as to the facts or their interpretation, "the chief difficulty" which they would oppose to the theory of germ-plasm would be, "that we are here concerned with the influence of the *germ-plasm* of the sperm-cell on a tissue of another plant which only constitutes *a part* of this plant." In other words, Weismann now freely entertains the possibility of a direct action of germ-plasm on the somatic tissues, even though these belong to another individual! Thus he now concedes the only point for the establishment of which I adduced the phenomena of xenia, in Chapter III: the whole of one side of that "reciprocal action between the sphere of germinal-substance and the sphere of body-substance," which I contended for on pp. 76-85, is now conceded; and although it is the less important side, its surrender goes far to weaken the doctrine of a perpetual isolation of germinal-substance to a "sphere" of its own. If we suppose that the germinal substance of one organism may thus directly act upon the somatic tissues of another, and that changed conditions of life are able to produce simultaneously an acquired character in the soma and a precisely identical character as congenital in the germ (pp. 129-30), we are plainly inviting ourselves to abandon the complex explanation of living material in "two kinds," where one is capable in all sorts of ways of communicating with the other, while the possibility of any reciprocal action is excluded. For the simpler hypothesis of living material as all of one kind encounters no such antinomies. So long as one kind of this material was supposed to be as distinct from the other as a parasite is distinct from its host, there was not so much to choose between the theory of germ-plasm and that of gemmules in this respect of simplicity. But the more that the former theory has had to be adjusted to facts, the greater has its complexity become, until now its own author is obliged to make so many additional assumptions for the purpose of mantaining it, that we begin to wonder how long it can continue to support the weight of its accumulating difficulties.

So much for the main modifications which have this year been made in Weismann's postulate of the perpetual continuity of germ-plasm. We must next consider the changes which he has effected in his companion postulate of the absolute stability of germ-plasm.

Weismann's Theory of Evolution (1893).

Of far more importance than any of the alterations which Professor Weismann has recently made in his theory of heredity, are those whereby he has modified his sequent theory of evolution. For while, as we have just seen, his work on *The Germ-plasm* leaves the former theory substantially unaltered,—although largely added to in matters of detail,—it so profoundly modifies the latter that careful readers will find no small difficulty in ascertaining how much of it has been allowed to remain. I will consider only the main modifications, and these I will take separately.

It will be remembered that one distinctive feature in Weismann's theory of evolution has hitherto been, that the unicellular organisms differ from the multicellular in the following important particulars.

1. There being no division in unicellular organisms between germ-cells and somatic-cells, there is no possibility in them of the occurrence of amphimixis.

2. Consequently, there is no possibility in them of congenital variations, in the sense that these occur in multicellular organisms.

3. Hence the only causes of individual variation and of the origin of species in the unicellular organisms are the Lamarckian factors, just as in the multicellular the only cause of these things is natural selection.

4. Hence, also, the unicellular organisms are potentially immortal, while the multicellular have acquired mortality for certain adaptive reasons.

But now, with the exception of No. 4, all these positions have been abandoned. For, chiefly on account of the beautiful researches of Maupas, Weismann has come to perceive that no real distinction can be drawn between an act of sexual union in the multicellular organisms, and an act of conjugation in the unicellular. Amphimixis, therefore, is now held by him to occur equally in both these divisions of organic nature, with the consequence that the Protozoa and Protophyta owe their individual variations, and therefore the origin of their innumerable species, as exclusively to the action of natural selection as is the case with the Metazoa and Metaphyta. In fact, the term "amphimixis" has been coined in express relation to these very points.

It will be seen, however, that this important change of view merely postpones the question as to the origin of amphimixis, if the object of this process be that which Weismann supposes—viz., the providing of material in the way of congenital variations on which natural selection can act. Therefore he is obliged to assume that there now are, or once have been, organisms of a less organized character than even the lowest of the unicellular forms—organisms, that is to say, which possess no nucleus, but are wholly composed of undifferentiated bioplasm. These most primitive organisms it must have been that were not subject to any process of natural selection, but, in virtue of an exclusive action of the Lamarckian factors upon their protoplasmic substance, gave rise to individual variations which subsequently gave rise to a unicellular progeny—when the process of natural selection was immediately inaugurated, and thereafter entirely superseded the Lamarckian factors. Or, to state the matter in Weismann's own words:—

> My earlier views on unicellular organisms as the source of individual differences, in the sense that each change called forth in them by external influences, or by use and disuse, was supposed to be hereditary, must therefore be dismissed to some stage less distant from the origin of life. I now believe that such reactions under external influences can only obtain in the lowest organisms which are without any distinction between nucleus and cell-body. All variations which have arisen in them, by the operation of any causes whatever, must be inherited, and their hereditary individual variability is due to the direct influence of the external world.... If I am correct in my view of the meaning of conjugation as a method of amphimixis, we must believe that all unicellular organisms possess it, and that it will be found in numerous low organisms, in which it has not yet been observed[53].

It is not very clear, at first sight, how Professor Weismann, after having thus abandoned the propositions 1, 2, and 3, as above stated, manages to retain his former view as given in No. 4. Nevertheless he does so, by representing that a unicellular organism, even though it present such a considerable degree of organization as we meet with in the higher Protozoa, still resembles a germ-cell of a multicellular organism, in that it consists of all the essential constituents of a germ-cell, including germ-plasm in its nucleus. And inasmuch as a germ-cell is potentially immortal, so it must be with a unicellular organism; in the one case, as in the other, the design of the structure is that its contained germ-plasm shall fuse with the germ-plasm contained in the nucleus of another individual cell, when the life of both will be preserved. For my own part, however, I cannot see that in either case the *cell*, as distinguished from its contained *germ-plasm*, is thus shown to be potentially immortal. On the contrary, it appears to me a mere accident of the case that in a unicellular organism the immortal substance (germ-plasm) is contained in a single cell, which is at the same time a *free* cell, and, as such, is denominated an "organism." We might just as well call a germ-cell an "organism," whether as an ovum it happens to be embedded in a mass of somatic-cells, or as a locomotive spermatozoon it happens to be free. In fact Weismann himself appears to recognize this. But, if so, it is surely a distinction without a difference to say that unicellular organisms are immortal, while multicellular are mortal. For in neither case is the organism immortal, while in both cases it is the germ-plasm (i.e., the substance of heredity) that is so. Where the cell containing the germ-plasm happens to be a free cell, it is called an "organism"; but whether it be a germ-cell or a protozoan, it alike ceases to be a cell when it has given origin to a multitude of other cells, whether these happen to be other germ-cells (*plus* somatic-cells) or other protozoan cells. In short, *quâ* cell, all cells are mortal: it is only the substance of heredity which some cells contain that can be said, in any sense of the term, to be immortal. For the immortality in question does not belong to unicellular organisms as such, but to the germ-plasm which they contain. And from this it follows that, as the immortality of germ-plasm is one and the same thing as the continuity of germ-plasm, by alleging an immortality as belonging to the unicellular organisms, Weismann is merely restating his fundamental postulate. Hence, also, he is but denying, in a somewhat round-about way, the occurrence of spontaneous generation.

I conclude, therefore, that his sole remaining distinction between the unicellular and the multicellular organisms is but illusory, or unreal. And, with regard to the great change which he has thus effected in his system by expressly abolishing all the other distinctions, I have only to say that in my opinion he has thereby greatly improved his system. For he has thus relieved it of all the formidable difficulties which he had needlessly created for himself, and which I have already enumerated in the foregoing pages (88-89). In his ever-shifting drama of evolution the unicellular organisms have left the stage *en masse*, and, so far as they are concerned, we are all as we were before the curtain rose.

But of even more importance than this fundamental change of view with regard to the unicellular organisms, is a further and no less fundamental change with regard to the multicellular. That such is the case will immediately become apparent by a simple statement of the fact, that Weismann has now expressly surrendered his postulate of the absolute stability of germ-plasm!

We have already seen that, even in the first volume of his *Essays*, there were some passages which gave an uncertain sound with regard to this matter. But as they seemed attributable to mere carelessness on the part of their author, after quoting a sample of them, I showed it was necessary to ignore such inconsistent utterances—necessary, that is, for the purpose of examining the theory of germ-plasm as even so much as a logically coherent system of ideas[54]. For we have seen that if any doubt were to be entertained touching the *absolute* stability of germ-plasm "since the first origin of sexual propagation," a corresponding measure of doubt would be cast on Weismann's theory of congenital variation as *solely* due to amphimixis, with the result that his whole theory of evolution would be similarly rendered dubious. Since then, however, he has gone very much further in this direction. First, in reply to Professor Vines he says (1890):—

> I am at present inclined to believe that Professor Vines is correct in questioning whether sexual reproduction is the only factor which maintains Metazoa and Metaphyta in a state of variability. I could have pointed out in the English edition of my "Essays" that my views on this point had altered since their publication; my friend Professor de Bary, too early lost to science, had already called my attention to those parthenogenetic Fungi which Professor Vines justly cites against my views; but I desired, on grounds already mentioned, to undertake no alteration in the essays[55].

Next, in his essay on *Amphimixis* (1892), there are several passages to somewhat the same effect; while, lastly, in his *Germ-plasm* (1893), the fundamental postulate in question is, as I have said, expressly surrendered. For example, we have in the following words the final conclusions of his recent arguments. Speaking of amphimixis, he says:—

> *It is not the primary cause of hereditary variation.* By its means those specific variations which already exist in a species may continually be blended in a fresh manner, but it is incapable of giving rise to new variations, even though it often appears to do so.... *The cause of hereditary variation must lie deeper than this. It must be due to the direct effects of external influences on the biophores and determinants.*[56]

These quotations are enough to show that Weismann has now abandoned his original theory of congenital variations being exclusively due to amphimixis, and adopts in its stead the precisely opposite view—viz., that the origin of all such variations must be ascribed to the direct influence of causes acting on germ-plasm from without. Up to the present year the very essence of the whole Weismannian theory of evolution has been that, owing to the stability of germ-plasm since the first origin of sexual propagation, "the origin of hereditary individual variations cannot indeed be found in the higher organisms, the Metazoa and Metaphyta; but is to be sought for in the lowest—the unicellular organisms," because "the formation of new species, which among the lower Protozoa could be achieved without amphigony, could only be attained by means of this process in the Metazoa and Metaphyta. It was only in this way that hereditary individual differences could arise and persist[57]."

But about the beginning of the present year we have this fundamental doctrine directly contradicted in such words as:—

> *The origin of a variation* is equally independent of selection and amphimixis, and is due to the constant occurrence of slight inequalities of nutrition in the germ-plasm[58].

This complete reversal of his previous doctrine brings Weismann into line with Darwin, who long ago gave very good reasons for the following conclusion:—

> Those authors who, like Pallas, attribute all variability to the crossing either of distinct races, or to distinct individuals belonging to the same race but somewhat different from each other, are in error; as are those authors who attribute all variability to the mere act of sexual union [*amphimixis*][59].

And again:—

> These several considerations alone render it probable that variability of every kind is directly or indirectly caused by changed conditions of life. Or, to put it under another point of view, if it were possible to expose all the individuals of a species during many generations to absolutely uniform conditions of life, there would be no variability[60].

Hence, Darwin was disposed to find the main, if not the only, causes of congenital variations in circumstances depending for their efficacy on the *instability* of what Weismann calls germ-plasm. And the noteworthy fact is, that Weismann has now adopted this view, to the destruction of his originally fundamental postulate touching the *stability* of germ-plasm since the first origin of sexual propagation.

By such a right-about-face manœuvre, Weismann has placed his critics in a somewhat difficult position. For, in the first place, it is only towards the close of *The Germ-plasm* that the manœuvre is executed, and then only in a few sentences such as I have just quoted—italicized, it is true, but otherwise so slightly emphasized that, as Professor Hartog has observed, no one of his reviewers has noticed it[61]. In the second place, he nowhere expressly recognizes the effects upon his theory of evolution, which necessarily follow from the change. And, lastly, the manner in which he endeavours to underpin that theory after having thus removed its logical foundation in his former postulate of the absolute stability of germ-plasm, is so peculiar that it is hard to epitomize his reasoning with due regard to brevity.

Speaking for myself, I can only say that my first impulse, after reading the sentences above quoted, was to cancel the whole of Chapter IV, as well as all those parts of Chapters I and III where the Weismannian theory of evolution is alluded to; and then to start anew with a bare statement that this theory had now been wholly discarded by its author. But after due consideration it seemed desirable to leave the criticism as it was originally written, not only on account of the reasons already stated in the Preface, but still more because I found it would be impracticable to start a new criticism of the greatly modified theory of evolution without introducing many and lengthy parts of the old one, for the purpose of showing how the most recent theory had been arrived at. Hence, seeing that my previous criticism was far from having been rendered obsolete by the large changes which had taken place in Weismann's system of theories, I concluded that it was best to retain what I had written, and add the present paragraphs for the purpose of dealing exclusively with the changes in question.

In now proceeding to do this, I think it is needless to occupy space by giving the reasons which have caused Weismann thus to abandon his doctrine of the universal stability of germ-plasm since the first origin of sexual propagation, and to substitute the precisely opposite doctrine of its universal instability. It is enough to say that these reasons all arise by way of logical necessity from the further working out in *The Germ-plasm* of his theory of heredity—or, more correctly, from the additions which he has there made to his previous views on the mechanism of heredity. Thus he has reversed his former doctrine touching the absolute stability of germ-plasm, not so much on account of any of the general considerations or particular facts which I have adduced against it in Chapter IV, as because it would not tally with the recent additions which he has made to other parts of his system. Any one who cares to follow this matter will find the reasons in question fully and lucidly stated in Chapter XIV of *The Germ-plasm*[62].

It is of more importance to consider the means whereby Weismann seeks to save his theory of evolution after he has thus removed its foundation in his former postulate of the absolute stability of germ-plasm. As far as I can understand, he seeks to do so as follows.

In the first place, it must be noted that after his changes of view with regard to polar bodies, unicellular organisms, and the significance of sexual reproduction, nothing remains of his original theory of evolution save what he can manage to retain of his original theory of variation as due to amphimixis. But, as we have just seen, he has surrendered this latter theory also. Therefore, at first sight it appears that no part of the former can possibly remain. Beginning at the apex, he has removed, stone by stone, his doctrine of descent, and, on arriving at its fundamental postulate—the absolute stability of germ-plasm—simply turns it upside down. Surely, therefore, it may be thought, there is here as complete a destruction as well could be of all this side of Weismann's system. Such, however, he endeavours to show is not the case. He regards it as still possible to retain so much of his theory of descent as is presented by what he can save of his theory of variation, thus:—

Although he now represents that the *instability* of germ-plasm is such that in *no* case can amphimixis have had anything to do with the *origin* of congenital variations, he continues to regard the *stability* of germ-plasm sufficiently great to necessitate, in *all* cases, the occurrence of amphimixis in order to promote the *development* of congenital variations. In other words, notwithstanding that he now thinks all congenital variations

73

must be begun by external conditions acting directly on an unstable germ-plasm, he also thinks that the *amount* of variation thus produced is likely to be exceedingly minute, and must therefore be increased by subsequent amphimixis in order to fall within the range of natural selection. So that, although powerless to initiate congenital variation, amphimixis must still play an indispensable part in the process of evolution, as in all cases a necessary condition to the occurrence of natural selection. External conditions first cause slight changes in the determinants of a species; but these are so slight that they have to be augmented by amphimixis before they constitute material on which natural selection can act, and hence before they can become of any significance either in ontogeny or phylogeny.

Such, I take it, is what Professor Weismann would now have us to understand; for otherwise I should have expected from him as frank a surrender of his theory of evolution (or the remnant thereof in his theory of variation) as he has made of its fundamental postulate. But, if such is his meaning, I may mention the reasons which appear to me to render it nugatory.

In the first place, it is evident that in thus minimizing the possible range of congenital variation due to the action of external conditions on a non-absolutely stable substance of heredity, Weismann is making a wholly gratuitous assumption, for the sole purpose of saving what remains of his theory of evolution—i. e., the doctrine of the immense importance of amphimixis.

We have already seen in the foregoing chapter that his original assumption of the *absolute* stability of germ-plasm was a gratuitous one, made for the purpose of supplying a foundation for constructing his theory of evolution. But still more gratuitous is the assumption which he has now substituted, for the purpose of saving as much of this theory as is left—the assumption, namely, that germ-plasm, although universally unstable, nevertheless everywhere presents only a certain low degree of instability, which serves to accommodate his modified theory of heredity on the one hand, and all that is possible of his previous theory of evolution on the other. His original assumption, untenable though it was, furnished at least a logical basis for the necessary conclusion that amphimixis was the only possible cause of congenital variations. But there is not so much as any logical sequence in the now substituted assumption, that (A) all congenital variations are ultimately due to the *universal instability* of germ-plasm, and (B) that nevertheless they are all more proximately due to such *a high degree of stability* of germ-plasm as necessitates amphimixis as the only means whereby variations can be made "perceptible." These statements are as independent of one another as any two statements can well be; and, therefore, if the second of them is to be substantiated, it can only be so by some totally distinct line of reasoning. The first statement does not even tend to suggest the second; in fact it tends to suggest the precise contrary. For, obviously, there is nothing in the logic of the matter to show why, if all congenital variations depend for their origin on the instability of germ-plasm, such instability must nevertheless be always so slight that the variations due to it must afterwards depend on amphimixis for their development to the point where they become "perceptible." As above indicated, it is surely little short of absurd thus to assume that a universally unstable germ-plasm universally presents only that particular degree of instability which will serve to accommodate Professor Weismann's newer theory of heredity, and at the same time to save thus much of his previous theory of evolution.

But now, in the second place, not only is this assumption wholly gratuitous, but there are many considerations which render it in the highest degree improbable, while there are not wanting facts which appear to demonstrate that it is false. For, unquestionably, most of the considerations which have already been advanced in the preceding chapter against the assumption of an absolute stability of germ-plasm, are here equally available against the assumption of an imperceptibly small amount of instability[63]. Similarly, all the facts there given with regard to the a-sexual origin of species—and even genera—of parthenogenetic organisms, bud-variation[64], &c., amply demonstrate that congenital variations due to the instability of germ-plasm alone, or apart from amphimixis, are sometimes enormous. Hence, we cannot accept the gratuitous suggestion that in all other cases they are too insignificant to count for anything till they have been augmented by amphimixis, even although we may be prepared to agree that amphimixis is probably one important factor in the production of congenital variations. What degree of importance it presents in this connexion, however, we have not at present any means of determining; all we can conclude with certainty is, that in some cases it is demonstrably very much less than Weismann supposes, while it is extremely improbable that it is ever in any case the sole and necessary antecedent to the operation of natural selection.

This extreme improbability is shown, not only by what I have already said in the previous chapter, and need not here repeat; but likewise by the "several considerations" which Darwin has adduced with regard to this very point, and which, as he says, "alone render it probable that variability of every kind is directly or indirectly caused by changed conditions of life," with the consequence that "those authors who attribute all variability to the mere act of sexual union are in error." I have already quoted these words further back in the present chapter, in order to show that by now attributing the *origin* of all congenital variations to the direct action of external conditions, Weismann has brought himself into line with Darwin so far as this fundamental point of doctrine is concerned. But I here re-quote the words in order to show that by further attributing the *development* of congenital variations "to the mere act of sexual union," Weismann is again falling out of line with Darwin. So to speak, he first performs a right-about-face movement as regards his original position towards the "stability of germ-plasm," and immediately afterwards makes a half-turn back again. Now, it is this half-turn to which I object as unwarranted in logic and opposed to fact.

In a previous chapter (pp. 66-7) I presented to him the dilemma, that germ-plasm must be either absolutely stable or else but highly stable, and that in the former case his theory of amphimixis as the sole cause of congenital variations would be valid, while in the latter case the theory would collapse. But it did not then occur to me that Weismann might seek a narrow seat between the horns of this dilemma, by representing that germ-plasm is universally unstable up to a certain very low degree of instability—viz., exactly that degree which is required for starting a congenital variation by means of external causes, without its being possible for the variation to become perceptible unless afterwards increased by means of amphimixis. And now that this extremely sophistical position has been adopted, I cannot see any imaginable reason for adopting it other than a last endeavour to save as much as possible of his former theory of evolution. There can be nothing in the nature of things thus to limit, within the narrowest possible range, the instability of a universally unstable germ-plasm—distributed, as this most complex of known substances is, throughout all species of plants and animals, and exposed to inconceivably varied conditions of life in all quarters of the globe. And these considerations are surely of themselves enough to dispose of the assumption as absurd, without again rehearsing the facts of congenital variation which definitely prove it to be false.

Conclusion.

For reasons stated at the commencement of this chapter, I have restricted its subject-matter almost exclusively to a consideration of the more fundamental changes which Professor Weismann has wrought in his general system of theories by the publication of his most recent works. In other words, I have purposely avoided considering those immensely elaborate additions to his theory of heredity which constitute by far the largest portion of his essays on *Amphimixis* and *The Germ-plasm*, and which have for their object an ideal construction of "the architecture of germ-plasm."

The fundamental changes to which allusion has just been made are as follows.

Professor Weismann has to a large extent abandoned his theory of polar bodies, and in my opinion would have done well had he taken a further step and surrendered the theory *in toto*.

Similarly, he has withdrawn his previous distinctions between the unicellular and multicellular organisms. The Protozoa and Protophyta are now included by him in the same category as the Metazoa and Metaphyta, as regards all matters of individual variation, reproduction, subjection to the law of natural selection, and so forth. The only difference which he continues to allege is the somewhat metaphysical one touching mortality and immortality. But I have given what appears to me sufficiently good reasons for ignoring this distinction; and therefore, as it seems to me, every one of Weismann's previous doctrines respecting unicellular organisms have vanished—very much to the benefit of his system as a whole.

By far the greatest change, however, which he has made in this general system is that which he has effected by surrendering the postulate of the absolute stability of germ-plasm. The rift in his lute which has been noticed with regard to this matter has now been widened to an extent which *does* prevent any further harping on the theme of evolution. It is true that Weismann endeavours to retain as far as possible the general character of his former postulate of the universal stability of germ-plasm, with the consequent "significance of sexual reproduction" as the sole cause of congenital variation. For although he now reverses both these doctrines by saying that germ-plasm is universally unstable, and that sexual reproduction is in no case the sole cause of congenital variation, he seeks at the same time to minimize the logical consequences of such reversal by making an ingenious assumption, the possibility of which I had not foreseen when writing the previous chapters. The assumption is, that although germ-plasm is universally unstable, the degree of its instability is everywhere restricted within the narrowest possible limits; so that sexual propagation is still necessary for the purpose of *developing* congenital variations to the point where they can fall within the range of natural selection, notwithstanding that they must all have been *originated* by external causes acting directly on a germ-plasm universally unstable within the narrow limits assumed. But clearly this assumption is arbitrary to the last degree, and, no less clearly, it is made by Weismann for the sole purpose of saving as much as he can of his previous theory of variation. His more recent speculations touching the mechanism of heredity are incompatible with his former view of amphimixis as the *sole* cause of congenital variations, and therefore he makes this arbitrary assumption for the purpose of representing that amphimixis may nevertheless still be regarded as a *necessary con-cause*. I need not here repeat what has so recently been said touching the sophistry of this assumption in theory, or the demonstrable falsity of it in fact. It is enough to remark, in conclusion, that the game is not worth the candle. It was originally well worth Weismann's while to sustain his fundamental postulate of the *absolute* stability of germ-plasm, because he was able to rear upon it his whole theory of evolution. But the only part of this theory which he has now left standing, or which he can now save by his newer postulate of a germ-plasm both stable and unstable at the same time, is his doctrine of variation. So to speak, it is his desire to reserve as much as is speculatively possible from the general ruin of his theory of descent, that causes him to go so far to attempt so little. For I cannot suppose that he himself will expect any of his readers to entertain so arbitrary, fanciful, and demonstrably false an assumption as the one in question. Surely it would have been better to have surrendered *in toto* this "Weismannian theory of variation," rather than to have attempted its rescue by means so plainly nugatory. It might still have been held that amphimixis plays a large and important part as one of the causes of variation, and therefore also as one of the factors of organic evolution. After having reversed his postulate of amphimixis being the sole cause of variability, and therefore having agreed with Darwin that "those writers are in error who attribute all variability to the mere act of sexual union," he might well have questioned Darwin's further statement as to its being "probable that variability of every kind is directly or indirectly caused by changed conditions of life." But by now assuming that variations due to any causes other than amphimixis must be "imperceptible" until they have been augmented by amphimixis, Weismann is shutting out, with a futile hypothesis, the important question as to whether, or how far, amphimixis really is a cause of variation. Observe, the case is not as it might have been were there no reasons assignable for the occurrence of sexual propagation, other than that of assisting in the production of congenital variations. The theory of "rejuvenescence," for example, is *prima facie* a more probable one than that which ascribes to sexual propagation the function of causing variability[65]; while Galton's hypothesis, which supposes the object of this form of propagation to be that of conserving the "germs" (= "determinants") of the phyla, has a good deal to say for itself[66]. Of course such alternative hypotheses touching "the significance of sexual reproduction" are not necessarily exclusive of one another: the process may subserve two or more adaptive purposes[67]. But he would be a bold man who, in the present state of our knowledge, could accept unreservedly the particular view of this process which Darwin so emphatically rejected; and I think he must be a biased man who could entertain for an instant the modification of this view which Weismann has now substituted.

Thus, the Weismannian theory of evolution has entirely fallen to pieces with the removal of its fundamental postulate—the absolute stability of germ-plasm. It only remains to mention once more the effects of this removal upon the other side of his system—viz., the companion postulate of the uninterrupted continuity of germ-plasm, with its superstructure in his theory of heredity.

Briefly, these effects are as follows:—

1. Germ-plasm ceases to be continuous in the sense of having borne a perpetual record of congenital variations from the first origin of sexual propagation.

2. On the contrary, as all such variations have been originated by the direct action of external conditions, the continuity of germ-plasm in this sense has been interrupted at the commencement of every inherited change during the phylogeny of all plants and animals, unicellular as well as multicellular.

3. But germ-plasm remains continuous in the restricted, though still highly important sense, of being the sole repository of hereditary characters of each successive generation, so that acquired characters can never have been transmitted to progeny "representatively," even although they have frequently caused those "specialized" changes in the structure of germ-plasm which, as we have seen, must certainly have been of considerable importance in the history of organic evolution.

4. By surrendering his doctrine of the *absolute* stability of germ-plasm on the one hand, and of its *perpetual*[68] continuity on the other, Weismann has greatly improved his theory of heredity. For, whatever may be thought of his recent additions to this theory in the way of elaborate speculation touching the ultimate mechanism of heredity, it is a great gain to have freed his fundamental postulate of the continuity of germ-plasm from the two further postulates which have just been mentioned, and the sole purpose of which was to provide a basis for his untenable theory of evolution.

5. In my opinion it only remains for him to withdraw the last remnant of his theory of evolution by cancelling his modified and even less tenable views on amphimixis, in order to give us a theory of heredity which is at once logically intact and biologically probable.

6. The theory of germ-plasm would then resemble that of stirp in all points of fundamental importance, save that while the latter leaves the question open as to whether acquired characters are ever inherited in any degree, the former would dogmatically close it, chiefly on the grounds which I have considered in Appendix II. It seems to me that in the present state of our knowledge it is more prudent to follow Galton in suspending our judgement with regard to this question, until time shall have been allowed for answering it by the inductive methods of observation and experiment.

7. Hence, in conclusion, we have for the present only to repeat what Weismann himself has said in one of the wisest of his utterances,—"The question as to the inheritance of acquired characters remains, whether the theory of germ-plasm be accepted or rejected."

It is now close upon twenty years that I accepted the substance of this theory under the name of stirp; and since that time the question as to the inheritance of acquired characters remains exactly where it was. No new facts, and no new considerations of much importance, have been forthcoming to assist us in answering it. Therefore, as already stated in the Preface, I intend to deal with this question hereafter as a question *per se*, or one which is not specially associated with the labours of Professor Weismann.

APPENDIX I:

ON GERM-PLASM.

As already stated in the text (p. 71), Weismann's general reasoning in support of his own theory of germ-plasm, as against Darwin's theory of gemmules in any form, admits of being reduced to arguments in favour of three propositions—viz., first, that there is no evidence of the transmission of somatogenetic characters; secondly, that the theory of pangenesis, which seeks to explain their supposed transmission, is "inconceivable"; and, thirdly, that its logical antithesis—the theory of germ-plasm—is so much less beset with difficulties, that by comparison it is simple, self-coherent, and offers a real, as distinguished from a "formal," explanation of the facts of heredity.

The first of these propositions will be discussed at considerable length in my next volume. The second and third propositions, however, may be dealt with here.

The following paragraph, which I shall quote sentence by sentence, sets forth the grounds on which Weismann bases the second proposition, namely, that any theory belonging to the order of pangenesis—i. e., which supposes the carriers of heredity ever to travel centripetally—is, from its very nature, inconceivable.

> At first sight this hypothesis seems to be quite reasonable. It is not only conceivable that particles might proceed from the somatic to the reproductive cells, but the very nutrition of the latter at the expense of the former is a demonstration that such a passage actually takes place. But a closer examination reveals immense difficulties. In the first place, the molecules of the body devoured are never simply added to those of the feeding individual without undergoing any change, but, as far as we know, they are really assimilated, that is, converted into the molecules of the latter. We cannot therefore gain much by assuming that a number of molecules can pass from the growing somatic cells into the growing reproductive cells, and can be deposited unchanged in the latter, so that, at their next division, the molecules are separated to become the somatic cells of the following generation[69].

The obvious answer to this is, that no one has ever supposed "gemmules" to be merely "*molecules*," in the chemical sense of this word; nor has any one ever imagined that they are "*devoured*" by the germ-cells into which they pass. Of course, if this were the case—i.e., if gemmules serve merely as *food* to the germ-cells—they would become disintegrated down even to their chemically molecular structure, and there would be an end of them as organized "carriers of heredity."

In the second place, it is asked:—

> How can such a process [i.e. the passage of gemmules into growing germ-cells] be conceivable, when the colony becomes more complex, when the number of somatic cells becomes so large that they surround the reproductive cells with many layers, and when at the same time, by an increasing division of labour, a great number of different tissues and cells are produced, all of which must originate *de novo* from a single reproductive cell?

Here, again, the obvious answer is, that no one has ever propounded such a statement. Far from supposing that "all the different cells and tissues of a complex organism must originate *de novo* from a *single* reproductive cell," the theory of pangenesis supposes the very contrary—viz., that somatic changes in the past history of the phyla have *not* thus originated in *any* reproductive cell. The idea of somatic changes originating in reproductive cells belongs to the theory of *germ-plasm*; but even this theory does not suppose all the great number of different cells and tissues which compose a complex organism to have ever originated *de novo* from a *single* reproductive cell.

The difficulty touching germ-cells becoming isolated, or buried, by the phylogenetic increase of somatic cells, is enforced in the immediately succeeding sentences, thus:—

> Each of these various elements [somatic cells] must, *ex hypothesi*, give up certain molecules to the reproductive cells; hence those which are in immediate contact with the latter would obviously possess an advantage over those which are more remote. If, then, any somatic cell must send the same number of molecules to each reproductive cell[70], we are compelled to suspend all known physical and physiological conceptions, and must make the entirely gratuitous assumption of an affinity on the part of the molecules for the reproductive cells. Even if we admit the existence of this affinity, its origin and means of control remain perfectly unintelligible if we suppose that it has arisen from differentiation of the complete colony. An unknown controlling force must be added to this mysterious arrangement, in order to marshal the molecules which enter the reproductive cell in such a manner that their arrangement corresponds with the order in which they must emerge as cells at a later period.

Now I do not see much force in the suggestion that those somatic cells which happen to be in immediate contact with germ-cells, "must obviously possess an advantage over those which are more remote." On the contrary, I do not see that mere proximity of one species of cell to another species within the same organism need have anything to do with the matter—still less that "we must suspend all physical and physiological conceptions," if we demur to the statement that it "obviously must." As for "physical conceptions," how many thousands of cases might not be pointed to among chemical and mechanical processes where contact or proximity are conditions of comparatively little importance? And as for "physiological conceptions," do we find that any part of the organism is affected by its distance, say, from the liver and kidneys, for getting rid of its effete products? Is it not rather the case that every gland in the body is wholly unaffected by its distance from any part of the body, in regard to its function of draining off the particular substances with which it is concerned? Why then should the reproductive gland constitute a conspicuous exception? Or how do we suspend all physiological conceptions, if we suppose that this gland resembles every other gland in being specialized to *secrete* a particular kind of "molecule," which, because thus specially *selected*, may be said to have for that gland a special "affinity"? If there are such things as gemmules, I do not see any violation of physiological analogies—still less an "entirely gratuitous assumption"—in supposing that they can be filtered out from all parts of the body by the sexual glands, and there aggregated as a special product to be discharged in the form of sexual elements[71].

But, it is further represented, "even if we admit the existence of this affinity, an unknown controlling force must be added to this mysterious arrangement, in order to marshal the molecules which enter the [growing] reproductive cell in such a manner that

80

their arrangement corresponds with the order in which they emerge as cells at a later period." Surely, however, for Weismann of all naturalists it ought not to be difficult to find this "unknown controlling force." For of all naturalists he is perhaps the most ready to invoke the agency of natural selection as sufficient to explain every case—actual or imaginable—of *adaptation*. Now, here is a case where natural selection, one would think, is positively bound to act—supposing that there be such things as gemmules. For, if "the carriers of heredity" are gemmules, it is evident that their mutual "affinities" must be adaptively "marshalled" at each step of phylogenetic evolution, before any further advance of such evolution can be possible. And I do not see anything more "inconceivable" in supposing the establishment of such mutual affinities step by step through natural selection, than in supposing any other course of adaptive development by similar means. For, as Darwin has well shown, while anticipating this particular objection to his theory,—"The assumed elective affinity of each gemmule for that particular cell which precedes it in due order of development is supported by many analogies." The analogies which he then gives are so numerous that I must here refer to his own discussion of the subject[72]—a discussion which is entirely ignored by Weismann.

Lastly, the principal ground, as far as I can see, which Weismann has for regarding Darwin's theory in any shape "inconceivable," is his own supposition that there is as complete an anatomical separation between the soma and its germ-cells as there is, for example, between the mammalian soma and these same cells when afterwards detached from the ovary and developing as foetuses *in utero*. In other words, the only connexion is supposed to be that of deriving nourishment by way of imbibition. But, as regards the germ-cell while still forming in the ovary or testicle, there is for this supposition no basis in fact. There is nothing in the histology of spermatogenesis that lends countenance to the supposition, while in the case of the ovum such histological evidence as we possess makes altogether against it. As Professor Vines has remarked:—

> It cannot be seriously maintained that the whole body of the embryo is developed solely from the germ-plasm of the ovum. On the contrary, since the embryo is developed from the whole of the nucleus and more or less of the cytoplasm of the ovum, it must be admitted that the non-germ-plasm of the ovum provides a large part of the material in embryogeny. It is an obvious inference that, under these circumstances, hereditary characters may be transmitted from the parent to the offspring, not only by the germ-plasm, but also by the somato-plasm, of the ovum[73].

Again, and apart from this consideration, it is now known that a very intimate network of protoplasmic fibres connects the cell-contents of cellular tissues, both in plants and animals. So that here we have another very possible means of communication between the germ-cells and the somatic-cells which together constitute a multicellular organism.

Therefore, in so far as histology can be trusted to constitute a basis for generalizations of this kind at all, it does not sustain the supposition that there can be no medium of communication between the general cellular tissues of an organism and its specially reproductive elements. On the contrary, the microscope is able to demonstrate possible roads of connexion—and this even upon Weismann's own view as to a specialized germinal substance which is restricted to the nucleus of an ovum. In short, the supposition as to an absolute anatomical separation between germ-plasm and somato-plasm is a deduction from Weismann's theory itself: it is not supported—it is discredited—by histological observation. Hence, it cannot be accepted as valid evidence in favour of the theory from which alone it is derived, or as a valid objection to the rival theory of pangenesis.

Once more, even if it were true that histology proves an absolute anatomical isolation on the part of germ-cells, it would still have remained unquestionable that there is no absolute *physiological* isolation. For, at least, the germ-plasm derives its nourishment from the soma in which it resides; and who shall say that the process of mere imbibition is not amply sufficient to admit of the passage of "gemmules"? Call them what we choose, the "carriers of heredity" must be so unimaginably small, that in relation to histological cells they must be as gnats to camels. Yet we know that even camels in the form of "migrating cells" of various kinds are able to pass through living membranes; and we also know that the microbes of syphilis can penetrate both ova and spermatozoa. Why then should it be deemed inconceivable that, where all such things can pass, gemmules can do so likewise?

Lastly, I have recently spoken of the detached condition of a ripe ovum *in utero*. Now it seems to me more "inconceivable" that such an ovum should be capable of announcing, as it were, to the walls of the uterus whether or not it is in a fertilized condition, than it is that, before quitting the ovary, it should have had some kind of physiological converse with its environing soma. Yet it is certain that, without any visible medium of communication, the impregnated ovum is able to inform the uterus that it is impregnated; and thereupon the uterus behaves towards that ovum in an altogether astonishing manner, such as it never displays towards an unimpregnated ovum. Of course various hypotheses may now be formed to account for this fact, seeing that no one can question it as a fact. But supposing that the fact could be questioned, with how much greater effect might it be argued that any communication between the ovum and its soma is even more antecedently incredible when the ovum is entirely free than when it is still contained within its ovary.

Now these, as far as I can find, are the only grounds for Weismann's repeated assertion that the theory of pangenesis in any form is "inconceivable." I have therefore endeavoured to show that this is too strong a statement. All the facts and considerations whereby he seeks to support it were present to the mind of Darwin; and, quite apart from any question of relative authority, I cannot avoid agreeing with Darwin that, whether or not the theory is true, at all events the "difficulties" attaching to it on these merely *a priori* grounds are not insuperable, or such as to render his "pet child" an unconceived monstrosity in logic, or a proved absurdity in science.

Be it understood, however, that I am not here defending the theory of pangenesis. I am investigating the theory of germ-plasm; and it is because Weismann seeks to sustain the latter by excluding the former as preposterous, that I have been obliged thus to consider the validity of his criticism. For the point to which I am leading is, that Weismann gains nothing in the way of support to his own theory by this disparagement of Darwin's, *unless he can show that the former supplies some more "conceivable" explanation touching the mechanism of heredity.* Now I am unable to see that he has shown this. What I do see is that his *a priori* argument from "inconceivability" cuts both ways, and that it makes at least as much against germ-plasm as it does against gemmules.

Therefore, having now considered what Weismann has said against the conceivability of gemmules on grounds of general reasoning, I shall proceed to show that quite as much—or even more—may be said in the way of a *tu quoque*. In other words, we have now finished with the second of the three propositions which we are examining (see p. 71), and proceed to our consideration of the third.

First of all, I do not see any greater difficulty in supposing that the "carriers of heredity" proceed centripetally from somatic-cells to germ-cells, than in supposing that they proceed centrifugally from the germ-cells to the somatic-cells which they are engaged in constructing. Nor do I see any more difficulty in imagining these "carriers of heredity" to be capable of constructing a new organism if they have first proceeded centripetally, and are thus severally representative of all parts of the parent organism *after its construction has been completed*, than I do if they have proceeded centrifugally, and are thus similarly representative of all parts of that organism *before its construction has been commenced*[74].

Similarly, it seems to me, whatever cogency there may be in Weismann's objection to Darwin's theory on the score that it must assume "an unknown controlling force in order to marshal the molecules," is equally great as regards his own. True, Weismann has a lot to say about the control which nucleo-plasm can exercise on cell-formation, and germ-plasm on marshalling successive stages of ontogeny; but all that this amounts to is a re-statement of the facts. Such a controlling force must be equally assumed by both theories; but in each alike there is an absence of any ghost of an explanation.

Again, whatever difficulty there may be in conceiving the transition of somatic substance, *mutatis mutandis* there must be an equal difficulty in conceiving the transition of germinal substance into somatic substance. Indeed, as far as I can see, the difficulty is even greater in the latter case than it is in the former. For the very essence of Weismann's view is that germ-plasm differs from all or any other "plasm" in origin or kind: germ-plasm, and germ-plasm alone, has been immortal, perpetually continuous, capable of indefinite self-multiplication, and so of differentiating itself into an endless number and variety of somatic tissues. But, according to Darwin's view, there is not, and never has been, any such fundamental difference between the essential nature of somatic elements, and the essential nature of sexual elements. On the contrary, it is supposed that both formative and formed material are one in kind—that all the cellular tissues of a multicellular organism, like the single cell of a unicellular organism, are *per se* endowed with the vital property of self-multiplication; and that whether this property finds its expression in normal growth, in abnormal increments of growth (such as tumours), in processes of repair, in the various forms of a-sexual reproduction, or in the more specialized form of sexual fertilization, there is everywhere an exhibition of one and the same capacity. Now, without going further than this contrast between the fundamental principles of the two theories, does it not become evident that the difficulty of conceiving a transition of A into A′ is at any rate no greater than that of conceiving a transition of A into B, where A is in both cases the formative substance, A′ this same substance in another stage of evolution (i.e., elaborated for the performance of some special function, but never so as to lose its original function A), while B is a substance which differs from A almost as much as a woven texture differs from the hands that weave it?

Once more, in all his arguments which are directed to prove the continuity of germ-plasm, Weismann nowhere seems to perceive the necessity of arguing the correlative hypothesis—viz., that of the discontinuity of somato-plasm. Yet, as Professor Vines has remarked, it is as incumbent on him to disprove any possible continuity on the part of somato-plasm, as it is to prove a perpetual continuity on the part of germ-plasm. And here I am disposed to go further than Professor Vines has gone; for it appears to me even *more* incumbent on Weismann to argue a discontinuity on the part of somato-plasm, than it is on him to argue a continuity on the part of germ-plasm.

This must be immediately apparent if we remember that, unless the discontinuity of somato-plasm be assumed, the theory of the continuity of germ-plasm in telluric time (as distinguished from eternity) becomes identical in form with all those theories of heredity to the family of which pangenesis belongs. All these theories go upon the assumption that living material has been continuous in telluric time—i.e., always derived from pre-existing material of the same kind; but they embody the further assumption that *all* living material *is* material of the same kind—i.e., everywhere presents the same fundamental properties. Weismann's theory on the other hand, while adopting the first assumption, rejects the second; and assumes in its stead that living material exists in "two kinds," only one of which has been continuous, while the other is discontinuous—being, in fact, formed anew at each ontogeny. Therefore, to my mind, it seems more needful to argue the point wherein his theory differs from these other theories of heredity, than it is to argue the point wherein it agrees with them. We look to him for a proof of the discontinuity of somato-plasm much more than we do for a proof of the continuity of germ-plasm. Now the only proof that he has to give of the discontinuity of somato-plasm—or, in other words, that the self-multiplication of somatic cells cannot take place unless the nucleus of each contains a self-multiplying idio-plasm derived from the nucleus of a germ-cell—is the non-transmissibility of somatogenetic characters. Here, however, there is an obvious equivoque. For his only test of characters as somatogenetic and blastogenetic consists in observing whether or not they are inherited: if they are inherited, he says they are blastogenetic: if they are not inherited, he says they are somatogenetic. But this is manifestly circular reasoning, so long as the question in debate is as to the truth of his theory. What we require in proof of the distinguishing feature of that theory—i.e., the discontinuity of the hypothetical somato-plasm—is not merely the obvious fact that some characters are inherited while others are not, but independent proof that inherited and non-inherited characters correspond to a continuity of germ-plasm on the one hand, and a discontinuity of somato-plasm on the other. He shows us, indeed, what was well known before, that characters developed during the lifetime of the individual are seldom (if ever) inherited, while characters developed during the lifetime of the species are always inherited. Obviously, however, this fact is no proof of the assumed correlation just mentioned, because, as Darwin has clearly pointed out, it may very well be due to the much shorter time which has been allowed for what may be termed the impress of heredity. Therefore, supposing (with Darwin and others) that living material is all of one kind, and continuous, the fact on which Weismann relies admits of being explained without resorting to his more complex supposition of living material in two kinds, the one perpetually continuous, and the other interrupted at each ontogeny.

For these reasons it appears to me that, so far as the argument from "inconceivability" is concerned, it makes at least as much against the theory of germ-plasm as it does against the theory of pangenesis; and, therefore, that no argumentative advantage is gained from its use by Weismann. The truth probably is that, *whatever* the mechanism of heredity may actually be, it is at once so minute and so complex that its action is "inconceivable," or, more correctly, unimaginable. Be it again understood, therefore, that I am not arguing in favour of pangenesis. I am merely criticising what appears to me an unsound argument in favour of germ-plasm. All this general or merely *a priori* reasoning with regard to inconceivability is, as I have attempted to show, as available on the one side as on the other, and so fails to yield any observable advantage to either.

In conclusion it must be noticed, that Weismann now appears to have himself perceived the grave difficulties which lie against his antithesis between a hypothetical "germ-plasm" and a hypothetical "somato-plasm," notwithstanding that the former becomes converted into the latter at each ontogeny. At any rate, he allows that Vines' criticism upon this head is sound. But he is strongly of the opinion that, by means of a later emendation of his theory as originally published, he has succeeded in obviating these difficulties *in toto*. For my own part, as already several times observed in the text, I cannot in the least perceive that such is the case; and therefore I will quote *in extenso* what he has said in answer to Professor Vines. It will be seen that his newer emendation of the theory consists in substituting for his original "somato-plasm" two substances, which are called respectively "somatic idio-plasm" and "cytoplasm." And it is by means of this substitution that he thinks he has, in some way or another, overcome the contradiction involved in the doctrine (and, as it still seems to me, the essential doctrine of his whole theory of heredity) that "germ-plasm" becomes converted into "somato-plasm" during the course of every ontogeny. The following, at any rate, is his latest utterance upon the subject:—

I believe that the objections which Professor Vines makes to my theory of the continuity of germ-plasma rest solely on an unintentional confusion of my ideas, as he compares the opinions expressed in the second essay with those of the later ones, with which they do not tally. I will endeavour to make this clear. In this second essay (1883) I contrasted the body (soma) with the germ-cells, and explained heredity by the hypothesis of a "Vererbungs-substanz" in the germ-cells (in fact the germ-plasma), which is transmitted without breach of continuity from one generation to the next. I was not then aware that this lay only in the nucleus of the ovum, and could therefore contrast the entire substance of the ovum with the substance of the body-cells, and term the latter "somato-plasm." In Essay IV (1885) I had arrived, like Strasburger and O. Hertwig, at the conviction that the nuclear substance, the chromatin of the nuclear loops, was the carrier of heredity, and that the body of the cell was nutritive but not formative. Like the investigators just named, I transferred the conception of idio-plasm, which Nägeli had enunciated in essentially different terms, to the "Vererbungs-substanz" of the ovum-nucleus, and laid down that the nuclear chromatin was the idio-plasm not only of the ovum but of every cell, that it was the dominant cell-element which impressed its specific character upon the originally indifferent cell-mass. From then onwards, I no longer designated the cells of the body simply as "somato-plasm," but distinguished, on the one hand, the idio-plasm or "Anlagen-plasma" of the nucleus from the cell-body or "Cytoplasma," and, on the other, the idio-plasm of the ovum-nucleus from that of the somatic cell-nucleus; I also for the future applied "germ-plasm" to the nuclear idio-plasm of ovum and spermatozoon, and "somatic idio-plasm" to that of the body cells (e.g., p. 184). The embryogenesis rests, according to my idea, on alterations in the nuclear idio-plasm of the ovum, or "germ-plasm"; on p. 186, et seq., is pictured the way in which the nuclear idio-plasm is halved in the first cell-division, undergoing regular alterations of its substance in such a way that neither half contains all the hereditary tendencies, but the one daughter-nucleus has those of the ectoblast, the other those of the entoblast; the whole remaining embryogenesis rests on a continuation of this process of regular alterations of the idio-plasm. Each fresh cell-division sorts out tendencies which were mixed in the nucleus of the mother-cell, until the complete mass of embryonic cells is formed, each with a nuclear idio-plasm which stamps its specific histological character on the cell.

I really do not understand how Professor Vines can find such remarkable difficulties in this idea. The appearance of the sexual cells generally occurs late in the embryogeny; in order, then, to preserve the continuity of germ-plasm from one generation to the next, I propound the hypothesis that in segmentation it is not *all* the germ-plasm (i. e., idio-plasm of the first ontogenetic grade) which is transformed into the second grade, but that a minute portion remains unaltered in one of the daughter-cells, mingled with its nuclear idio-plasm, but in an inactive state; and that it traverses in this manner a longer or shorter series of cells, till, reaching those cells on which it stamps the character of germinal cells, it at last assumes the active state. This hypothesis is not purely gratuitous, but is supported by observations, notably by the remarkable wanderings of the germinal cells of Hydroids from their original positions.

But let us neglect the probability of my hypothesis, and consider merely its logical accuracy. Professor Vines says:—"The fate of the germ-plasm of the fertilized ovum is, according to Professor Weismann, to be converted in part into the somato-plasm (!) of the embryo, and in part to be stored up in the germ-cells of the embryo. This being so, how are we to conceive that the germ-plasm of the ovum can impress upon the somato-plasm (!) of the developing embryo the hereditary character of which it (the germ-plasm) is the bearer? This function cannot be discharged by that portion of the germ-plasm of the ovum which has become converted into the somato-plasm (!) of the embryo, *for the simple reason that it has ceased to be germ-plasm*, and must therefore have lost the properties characteristic of that substance. Neither can it be discharged by that portion of the germ-plasm of the ovum which is aggregated in the germ-cells of the embryo, for under these circumstances it is withdrawn from all direct relation with the developing somatic-cells. The question remains without an answer." I believe myself to have answered this above. I do not recognize the somato-plasm of Professor Vines; my germ-plasm, or idio-plasm of the first ontogenetic grade, is not modified into the somato-plasm of Professor Vines, but into idio-plasm of the second, third, fourth, hundredth, &c. grade, and every one impresses its character on the cell containing it.

It may be dullness, but I confess that this does not appear to me an "answer" to Professor Vines' criticism. Even though "idio-plasm of the first ontogenetic grade" has to become "idio-plasm of the second, third, fourth, hundredth, &c. grade," before in each of the grades concerned it can give origin to the somatic-cells which are distinctive of that grade, I cannot see that it makes any difference (in relation to Vines' criticism) whether we speak of those cells as containing "somato-plasm," or as containing "somatic idio-plasm" of such and such a grade, *plus* "cytoplasm." For whether we thus follow Weismann's earlier terminology or his later, we are so far speaking about exactly the same thing, namely, the transformation of "germ-plasm" into all the constituent cells of the "soma." The difficulty is, in Vines' words above cited, "to conceive that the germ-plasm of the ovum can impress upon the somato-plasm of the developing embryo the hereditary characters of which it (the germ-plasm) is the bearer"; and Weismann says that this difficulty, which he acknowledges, can now be answered by substituting for his original statement that "germ-plasm" becomes changed into "somato-plasm," the statement that it is "idio-plasm" *derived* from "germ-plasm" which thus "impresses its character on the cell containing it." But, "as a matter of logical accuracy," there is surely here a distinction without a difference. For what is the difference between saying that germ-plasm "impresses" its character on the contents of *all* somatic cells considered collectively under the term "somato-plasm," and saying that every "ontogenetic grade" of germ-plasm "impresses" *its* character on *each* successive group of somatic cells considered severally under the term "idio-plasm" of such and such a grade? At best this newer terminology has reference merely to a superadded hypothesis touching the *mode*—or rather the *history*—of the transition in question: it does not affect the original and essential doctrine of the transition itself.

APPENDIX II:

ON TELEGONY.

A WIDELY different view, however, is taken by Mr. Herbert Spencer with regard to the theoretical interpretation of telegony. This, indeed, is precisely the opposite view to the one which is given in the text. For while I agree with Professor Weismann in holding that the facts of telegony (supposing them to be facts) are as compatible with the theory of germ-plasm as with that of gemmules, "physiological units," or any other theory which postulates a centripetal flow of the carriers of heredity from somatic-cells to germ-cells, Mr. Spencer is of the opinion that these facts are destructive of any theory which postulates a continuity in the substance of heredity—i.e., a centrifugal flow of the carriers of heredity. And, unquestionably, Mr. Spencer's view is the prevalent one. Therefore, seeing that his opinion is not only of weight *per se*, but is shared by the scientific world in general, I will here transcribe a somewhat lengthy discussion which I have recently held with him upon the subject.

In the *Contemporary Review* for March, Mr. Spencer wrote as follows:—

> We pass now to evidence not much known in the world at large, but widely known in the biological world, though known in so incomplete a manner as to be undervalued in it. Indeed, when I name it probably many will vent a mental pooh-pooh. The fact to which I refer is one of which record is preserved in the museum of the College of Surgeons, in the shape of paintings of a foal borne by a mare not quite thoroughbred, to a sire which was thoroughbred—a foal which bears the markings of the quagga. The history of this remarkable foal is given by the Earl of Morton, F.R.S., in a letter to the President of the Royal Society (read November 23, 1820). In it he states that wishing to domesticate the quagga, and having obtained a male, but not a female, he made an experiment.

>> I tried to breed from the male quagga and a young chestnut mare of seven-eighths Arabian blood, and which had never been bred from; the result was the production of a female hybrid, now five years old, and bearing, both in her form and in her colour, very decided indications of her mixed origin. I subsequently parted with the seven-eighths Arabian mare to Sir Gore Ouseley, who has bred from her by a very fine black Arabian horse. I yesterday morning examined the produce, namely, a two-year-old filly and a year-old colt. They have the character of the Arabian breed as decidedly as can be expected, where fifteen-sixteenths of the blood are Arabian; and they are fine specimens of that breed; but both in their colour and in the hair of their manes they have a striking resemblance to the quagga. Their colour is bay, marked more or less like the quagga in a darker tint. Both are distinguished by the dark line along the ridge of the back, the dark stripes across the fore-hand, and the dark bars across the back part of the legs[75].

Lord Morton then names sundry further correspondences. Dr. Wollaston, at that time President of the Royal Society, who had seen the animals, testified to the correctness of his description, and, as shown by his remarks, entertained no doubt about the alleged facts. But good reason for doubt may be assigned. There naturally arises the question— How does it happen that parallel results are not observed in other cases? If in any progeny certain traits not belonging to the sire, but belonging to a sire of preceding progeny, are reproduced, how is it that such anomalously-inherited traits are not observed in domestic animals, and indeed in mankind? How is it that the children of a widow by a second husband do not bear traceable resemblances of the first husband? To these questions nothing like satisfactory replies seem forthcoming; and, in the absence of replies, scepticism, if not disbelief, may be held reasonable.

There is an explanation, however. Forty years ago I made acquaintance with a fact which impressed me by its significant implications; and has, for this reason I suppose, remained in my memory. It is set forth in the *Journal of the Royal Agricultural Society*, vol. xiv. (1853), pp. 214 et seq., and concerns certain results of crossing English and French breeds of sheep. The writer of the translated paper, M. Malingié-Nouel, Director of the Agricultural School of La Charmoise, states that when the French breeds of sheep (in which were included "the *mongrel* Merinos") were crossed with an English breed, "the lambs present the following results. Most of them resemble the mother more than the father; some show no trace of the father." Joining the admission respecting the mongrels with the facts subsequently stated, it is tolerably clear that the cases in which the lambs bore no traces of the father were cases in which the mother was of pure breed. Speaking of the results of these crossings in the second generation "having seventy-five per cent. of English blood," M. Nouel says:—"The lambs thrive, wear a beautiful appearance, and complete the joy of the breeder.... No sooner are the lambs weaned than their strength, their vigour, and their beauty begin to decay.... At last the constitution gives way ... he remains stunted for life": the constitution being thus proved unstable or unadapted to the requirements. How, then, did M. Nouel succeed in obtaining a desirable combination of a fine English breed with the relatively poor French breeds?

He took an animal from "flocks originally sprung from a mixture of the two distinct races that are established in these two provinces [Berry and La Sologne]," and these he "united with animals of another mixed breed, ... which blended the Tourangelle and native Merino blood of" La Beauce and Touraine, and obtained a mixture of all four races "without decided character, without fixity, ... but possessing the advantage of being used to our climate and management."

Putting one of these "mixed-blood ewes to a pure New-Kent ram ... one obtains a lamb containing fifty-hundredths of the purest and most ancient English blood, with twelve and a-half hundredths of four different French races, which are individually lost in the preponderance of English blood, and disappear almost entirely, leaving the improving type in the ascendant.... All the lambs produced strikingly resembled each other, and even Englishmen took them for animals of their own country."

M. Nouel goes on to remark that when this derived breed was bred with itself, the marks of the French breeds were lost. "Some slight traces could be detected by experts, but these soon disappeared."

Thus we get proof that relatively pure constitutions predominate in progeny over much mixed constitutions. The reason is not difficult to see. Every organism tends to become adapted to its conditions of life; and all the structures of a species, accustomed through multitudinous generations to the climate, food, and various influences of its locality, are moulded into harmonious co-operation favourable to life in that locality: the result being that in the development of each young individual, the tendencies conspire to produce the fit organization. It is otherwise when the species is removed to a habitat of different character, or when it is of mixed breed. In the one case its organs, partially out of harmony with the requirements of its new life, become partially out of harmony with one another; since, while one influence, say of climate, is but little changed, another influence, say of food, is much changed; and, consequently, the perturbed relations of the organs interfere with their original stable equilibrium. Still more in the other case is there a disturbance of equilibrium. In a mongrel the constitution derived from each source repeats itself as far as possible. Hence a conflict of tendencies to evolve two structures more or less unlike. The tendencies do not harmoniously conspire; but produce partially incongruous sets of organs. And evidently where the breed is one in which there are united the traits of various lines of ancestry, there results an organization so full of small incongruities of structure and action, that it has a much-diminished power of maintaining its balance; and while it cannot withstand so well adverse influences, it cannot so well hold its own in the offspring. Concerning parents of pure and mixed breeds respectively, severally tending to reproduce their own structures in progeny, we may therefore say, figuratively, that the house divided against itself cannot withstand the house of which the members are in concord.

Now if this is shown to be the case with breeds the purest of which have been adapted to their habitats and modes of life during some few hundred years only, what shall we say when the question is of a breed which has had a constant mode of life in the same locality for ten thousand years or more, like the quagga? In this the stability of constitution must be such as no domestic animal can approach. Relatively stable as may have been the constitutions of Lord Morton's horses, as compared with the constitutions of ordinary horses, yet, since Arab horses, even in their native country, have probably in the course of successive conquests and migrations of tribes become more or less mixed, and since they have been subject to the conditions of domestic life, differing much from the conditions of their original wild life, and since the English breed has undergone the perturbing effects of change from the climate and food of the East to the climate and food of the West, the organizations of the horse and mare in question could have had nothing like that perfect balance produced in the quagga by a hundred centuries of harmonious co-operation. Hence the result. And hence at the same time the interpretation of the fact that analogous phenomena are not perceived among domestic animals, or among ourselves; since both have relatively mixed, and generally extremely mixed, constitutions, which, as we see in ourselves, have been made generation after generation, not by the formation of a mean between two parents, but by the jumbling of traits of the one with traits of the other, until there exist no such conspiring tendencies among the parts as cause repetition of combined details of structure in posterity.

Expectation that scepticism might be felt respecting this alleged anomaly presented by the quagga-marked foal, had led me to think over the matter; and I had reached this interpretation before sending to the College of Surgeons Museum (being unable to go myself) to obtain the particulars and refer to the records. When there was brought to me a copy of the account as set forth in the "Philosophical Transactions," it was joined with the information that there existed an appended account of pigs, in which a parallel fact had been observed. To my immediate inquiry— "Was the male a wild pig?"—there came the reply: "I did not observe." Of course I forthwith obtained the volume, and there found what I expected. It was contained in a paper communicated by Dr. Wollaston from Daniel Giles, Esq., concerning his "sow and her produce," which said that

> she was one of a well-known black and white breed of Mr. Western, the Member for Essex. About ten years since I put her to a boar of the wild breed, and of a deep chestnut colour, which I had just received from Hatfield House, and which was soon afterwards drowned by accident. The pigs produced (which were her first litter) partook in appearance of both boar and sow, but in some the chestnut colour of the boar strongly prevailed.
>
> The sow was afterwards put to a boar of Mr. Western's breed (the wild boar having been long dead). The produce was a litter of pigs some of which, we observed with much

surprise, to be stained and clearly marked with the chestnut colour which had prevailed in the former litter.

Mr. Giles adds that in a second litter of pigs, the father of which was of Mr. Western's breed, he and his bailiff believe there was a recurrence, in some, of the chestnut colour, but admits that their "recollection is much less perfect than I wish it to be." He also adds that, in the course of many years' experience, he had never known the least appearance of the chestnut colour in Mr. Western's breed.

What are the probabilities that these two anomalous results should have arisen, under these exceptional conditions, as a matter of chance? Evidently the probabilities against such a coincidence are enormous. The testimony is in both cases so good that, even apart from the coincidence, it would be unreasonable to reject it; but the coincidence makes acceptance of it imperative. There is mutual verification, at the same time that there is a joint interpretation yielded of the strange phenomenon, and of its non-occurrence under ordinary circumstances.

And now, in the presence of these facts, what are we to say? Simply that they are fatal to Weismann's hypothesis. They show that there is none of the alleged independence of the reproductive cells; but that the two sets of cells are in close communion. They prove that while the reproductive cells multiply and arrange themselves during the evolution of the embryo, some of their germ-plasm passes into the mass of somatic-cells constituting the parental body, and becomes a permanent component of it. Further, they necessitate the inference that this introduced germ-plasm, everywhere diffused, is some of it included in the reproductive cells, subsequently formed. And if we thus get a demonstration that the somewhat different units of a foreign germ-plasm permeating the organism, permeate also the subsequently-formed reproductive cells, and affect the structures of the individuals arising from them, the implication is that the like happens with those native units which have been made somewhat different by modified functions: there must be a tendency to inheritance of acquired characters.

My reply to this appeared in the April issue of the *Contemporary Review*, as follows:—

Influence on Progeny of a Previous Sire.

This is the last of the arguments which Mr. Spencer advances against the position of Professor Weismann. Alluding to the case of Lord Morton's mare, he represents that the phenomenon which it serves so well to illustrate—viz., the influence of a previous sire on the progeny of another by the same dam—is hopelessly at variance with the theory of germ-plasm. I cannot quite gather the explanation which he would give of this phenomenon, further than that in some way or another it betokens an immediate influence of the hereditary material of the male on the body-tissues ("somatic cells") of the female. And this is the view which is taken of the phenomenon by the Lamarckians in general. Yet, if we consider all that such an explanation involves, we shall find that it is a highly complex explanation, for it involves the following chain of hypotheses:—The first impregnation affects many, if not all, the somatic tissues of the mother by the germinal matter of the father; these tissues, in their turn, react on the maturing ova; this action and reaction is such that when one of the ova is afterwards fertilized by a different sire, the resulting offspring more or less resemble the preceding sire. Unfortunately, neither Weismann himself nor any of his followers, as far as I know, has hitherto published an opinion on the subject; but I imagine that his answer would be three-fold. First, he may question the fact. Secondly, even admitting the fact, he may say it is much more easy to explain it by supposing that the germ-plasm of the first sire has in some way or another become partly commingled with that of the immature ova, as well as with that of the mature one which it actually fertilizes; and, if so, it would naturally assert its influence on the progeny of a subsequent sire. Millions of spermatozoa must have been playing around the ovaries after the first copulation, and only one of them was needed to fertilize the mature ovum. It is not necessary to suppose that some of the others succeeded in penetrating any of the immature ova, while these were still embedded in the substance of their ovaries. It may be that the life of "ids" Is not commensurate with that of their containing spermatozoa. After the latter have perished and disintegrated, their ids may escape in thousands of millions, bathing in a dormant state the whole surfaces of both ovaries. And, if so, it is conceivable that when subsequent ova mature—i.e., come to the surface of their ovaries and rupture their follicles—these dormant ids adhere to their porous walls, through which they may pass. This may not seem a very probable explanation; but, at any rate, it is a less improbable one than that on which the Neo-Lamarckians would found an argument against the continuity of germ-plasm. For,—

Thirdly, is it not literally inconceivable that this Neo-Lamarckian explanation can be the true one? Can it be seriously contemplated that there is any such mechanism as the explanation must needs assume? If it is difficult to accept such a machinery as is supposed by the theory of pangenesis, whereby every cell in the body casts off "gemmules," which are the carriers of heredity from their respective tissues to the germinal elements, what are we to say of such a machinery as the following:—A machinery which distributes through the body of a female gemmules from the disintegrated spermatozoa of her mate; which distributes them *selectively*, so that they shall all eventually lodge in those tissue-cells of the female which correspond, part for part, with the tissue-cells of the male from which they were originally derived; which then insures that when a gemmule has thus reached its appropriate cell in the female body, it will thereupon modify the pre-existing gemmules in that cell, so that when they are shed and go to form the germinal contents of future ova, they endow the latter with the hereditary qualities of the male in question?

Such, it seems to me, is a fair statement of the whole case up to date. But I think it may be apposite now to publish the main results of an inquiry on which I have been engaged for the last three years.

First as to the facts. The investigations have been pursued on three different lines: (1) I raised discussions on the subject in the principal breeders' and fanciers' journals of this country, and also of America. (2) I entered into private correspondence with contributors of the largest experience, and also with professional and amateur breeders, fanciers, &c., who addressed me directly on the subject. (3) I started experiments with the varieties which these inquiries indicated as most likely to yield positive results. At present nothing need be said with regard to these experiments, because they are not sufficiently matured. But it is desirable to state the general upshot of the correspondence.

The principal result is to show that the phenomenon is of much less frequent occurrence than is generally supposed. Indeed, it is so rare that I doubt whether it takes place in more than one or two per cent. of cases. I must add, however, that nearly all my professional correspondents would deem this an absurdly low estimate. Most of them are quite persuaded that it is of frequent occurrence, many of them regard it as a general rule, while some of them go so far as to make a point of always putting a mare, a bitch, &c. to a good pedigree male in her first season, so that her subsequent progenies may be benefited by his influence, even though they be engendered by inferior sires. But I am certain that these estimates must be largely discounted in view of merely accidental resemblances, and still more on account of the prevalent belief upon the subject, which, where unquestioningly entertained, prevents anything like a critical estimate being formed.

But that the phenomenon does occur in some small percentage of cases there can be no reasonable doubt—as a result, I mean, of analysing the hundreds of cases which have now been submitted to me, especially with regard to dogs. One thoroughly well observed case occurring among pedigree animals is worth any number of slipshod statements, when precedent belief, inefficient isolation, exaggeration of memory, and so forth, have to be allowed for. On the present occasion space does not admit of giving such special instances, so I must ask it to be taken for granted that my evidence is enough to prove the fact of a previous sire asserting his influence on a subsequent progeny, although this fact is one of comparatively rare occurrence. It may be added that I have failed to find any good evidence of its ever occurring at all in the case of man. For although I have met with an alleged instance of a white woman, who, after having borne children to a negro husband, had a second family to a white one, in which some negro characteristics appeared, I have not been able to meet with any corroboration of this instance. I have made inquiries among medical men in the Southern States of America, where in the days of slavery it was frequently the custom that young negresses should bear their first children to their masters, and their subsequent children to negro husbands; but it never seems to have been observed, according to my correspondents, that these subsequent children were other than pure negroes. Such, however, was not the same case as the one above mentioned, but a reciprocal case; and this may have made a difference. If any reader should happen to know of another instance where a negro was the first husband, I hope he will inform me as to the result.

It has hitherto puzzled me why the phenomenon in question, since it does certainly occur in some cases, should occur so rarely as the above inquiries prove. But I think that Mr. Spencer's suggestion on this point is a valuable one, as it seems to present an excellent promise of solving the puzzle.

This suggestion, it will be remembered, is that when the first sire is of a relatively stable and also of a markedly different ancestral stock from the dam—e.g., of a different species, as in the case of Lord Morton's mare—there will be most likelihood of his impressing his ancestral characters on the progeny of the second sire[76]. And, as he remarks, it would indeed be an extraordinary coincidence if both the well-authenticated cases given in the College of Surgeons Catalogue should have conformed to his explanation by mere accident. To which I may add that the supposition of such an accidental coincidence would seem to be virtually excluded by the recent occurrence of yet a *third* case of exactly the same kind. This took place in the Zoological Gardens, where a wild ass of one species was the previous sire to a foal born of another species: the subsequent sire was of the same species as the mother, and his foal, born a few months ago, presented an unmistakable resemblance to the other species. A brief account of the particulars is given by Mr. Tegetmeier in the *Field* for December 14, 1892.

So much, then, for the facts. As regards their interpretation, it certainly seems to me that the one which I have supposed to be given by Weismann is less difficult of acceptance than the one which is given by the Lamarckians, as we have seen above. But it also seems to me that the latter explanation is not the only one available under the Lamarckian hypothesis. For, even under this hypothesis, there is no need to assume that the influence of the first sire is exerted on all the somatic tissues of the mother, and that these again reflect this influence on the ovum which is afterwards fertilized by the second sire. A mechanism that could effect all this may well be deemed impossible. But a much simpler explanation can be furnished by the Neo-Lamarckians, on lines similar to those upon which I have supposed that Weismann's explanation would run. For, on their common supposition that the substance of heredity is particulate, it matters not in the present connexion whether we suppose the particles to be ids or gemmules. Indeed, it is more in accordance with the hypothetical endowments of the latter than of the former, that they should be capable of penetrating the coats of an ovum, if they can survive the disintegration of their containing spermatozoön. Nevertheless, thus far it does not seem to me that any theory belonging to the family of pangenesis can gain any advantage over the theory of germ-plasm, by appealing to the fact of a previous sire sometimes affecting the progeny of a subsequent one. The case, however, is widely different if we turn from animals to plants, thus.

The advantage which any theory of gemmules seeks to gain over the theory of germ-plasm by an appeal to the fact in question, consists in supposing that the influence of the previous sire is exercised in the first instance on the somatic cells of the female. For this would prove that the germinal elements of the male are capable of communicating their hereditary qualities, not only by mixing with the germinal elements of the female (as in ordinary fertilization) but also by direct contact with the general tissues of the female. And this again would prove that the fundamental postulate of the theory of germ-plasm is erroneous—i.e., the postulate of the continuity of germ-plasm, or of its perpetual restriction to a "sphere" of its own. This, as all who are acquainted with the literature of the subject will at once perceive, would be a serious blow to the whole Weismannian system. But, as we have seen, the current Lamarckian interpretation of the fact in question involves the supposition of a physiological machinery so inconceivably complex that instead of serving to corroborate the theory of gemmules (or of physiological units) it would go to render that theory incredible[77].

If, however, we turn to plants, we find a considerable number of facts which unquestionably demonstrate the only point which this interpretation has been adduced to suggest. For these facts show that, in not a few cases, the germinal matter of pollen-grains is capable of asserting its influence beyond the ovules to the somatic tissues of the ovary, and even to the flower-stalk of the mother plant. Here, then, we have simple and conclusive evidence of the material of heredity exercising a direct influence on somatic tissues. How this well-known fact is to be met by the theory of germ-plasm is a question which does not seem to have thus far engaged the attention of Professor Weismann, or of any of his followers. For particulars touching this phenomenon, so highly important in its relation to the theory of germ-plasm, I cannot do better than refer to the eleventh chapter of Darwin's work on the "Variation of Animals and Plants under Domestication."

Again, in the *Contemporary Review* for May, Mr. Spencer wrote:—

In the essay to which this is a postscript, conclusions were drawn from the remarkable case of the horse and quagga there narrated, along with an analogous case observed among pigs. These conclusions have since been confirmed. I am much indebted to a distinguished correspondent who has drawn my attention to verifying facts furnished by the offspring of whites and negroes in the United States. Referring to information given him many years ago, he says:—"It was to the effect that the children of white women by a white father had been *repeatedly* observed to show traces of black blood, in cases when the woman had previous connexion with [i. e., a child by] a negro." At the time I received this information, an American was visiting me; and, on being appealed to, answered that in the United States there was an established belief to this effect. Not wishing, however, to depend upon hearsay, I at once wrote to America to make inquiries. Professor Cope of Philadelphia has written to friends in the South, but has not yet sent me the results. Professor Marsh, the distinguished palæontologist, of Yale, New Haven, who is also collecting evidence, sends a preliminary letter in which he says:—"I do not myself know of such a case, but have heard many statements that make their existence probable. One instance, in Connecticut, is vouched for so strongly by an acquaintance of mine, that I have good reason to believe it to be authentic."

That cases of the kind should not be frequently seen in the North, especially nowadays, is of course to be expected. The first of the above quotations refers to facts observed in the South during slavery days; and, even then, the implied conditions were naturally very infrequent. Dr. W. J. Youmans of New York has, on my behalf, interviewed several medical professors, who, though they have not themselves met with instances, say that the alleged result, described above, "is generally accepted as a fact." But he gives me what I think must be regarded as authoritative testimony. It is a quotation from the standard work of Professor Austin Flint, and runs as follows:—

A peculiar and, it seems to me, an inexplicable fact is, that previous pregnancies have

an influence upon offspring. This is well known to breeders of animals. If pine-blooded

mares or bitches have been once covered by an inferior male, in subsequent fecundations

the young are likely to partake of the character of the first male, even if they be afterwards

bred with males of unimpeachable pedigree. What the mechanism of the influence of the

first conception is, it is impossible to say; but the fact is incontestable. The same influence is observed in the human subject. A woman may have, by a second husband, children who resemble a former husband, and this is particularly well marked in certain instances by the colour of the hair and eyes. A white woman who has had children by a negro may subsequently bear children to a white man, these children presenting some of the unmistakable peculiarities of the negro race[78].

Dr. Youmans called on Professor Flint, who remembered "investigating the subject at the time his larger work was written [the above is from an abridgment], and said that he had never heard the statement questioned."

Some days before I received this letter and its contained quotation, the remembrance of a remark I heard many years ago concerning dogs, led to the inquiry whether they furnished analogous evidence. It occurred to me that a friend who is frequently appointed judge of animals at agricultural shows, Mr. Fookes, of Fairfield, Pewsey, Wiltshire, might know something about the matter. A letter to him brought various confirmatory statements. From one "who had bred dogs for many years" he learnt that—

> It is a well-known and admitted fact that if a bitch has two litters by two different dogs, the character of the first father is sure to be perpetuated in any litters she may afterwards have, no matter how pure-bred a dog may be the begetter.

After citing this testimony, Mr. Fookes goes on to give illustrations known to himself.

> A friend of mine near this had a very valuable Dachshund bitch, which most unfortunately had a litter by a stray sheep-dog. The next year her owner sent her on a visit to a pure Dachshund dog, but the produce took quite as much of the first father as the second, and the next year he sent her to another Dachshund with the same result. Another case:—A friend of mine in Devizes had a litter of puppies, unsought for, by a setter from a favourite pointer bitch, and after this she never bred any true pointers, no matter of what the paternity was.

These further evidences, to which Mr. Fookes has since added others, render the general conclusion incontestable. Coming from remote places, from those who have no theory to support, and who are some of them astonished by the unexpected phenomena, the agreement dissipates all doubt. In four kinds of mammals, widely divergent in their natures—man, horse, dog, and pig— we have this same seemingly anomalous kind of heredity made visible under analogous conditions. We must take it as a demonstrated fact that, during gestation, traits of constitution inherited from the father produce effects upon the constitution of the mother; and that these communicated effects are transmitted by her to subsequent offspring. We are supplied with an absolute disproof of Professor Weismann's doctrine that the reproductive cells are independent of, and uninfluenced by, the somatic cells; and there disappears absolutely the alleged obstacle to the transmission of acquired characters....

There is one other passage in Dr. Romanes' criticism—that concerning the influence of a previous sire on progeny—which calls for comment. He sets down what he supposes Weismann will say in response to my argument. "First, he may question the fact." Well, after the additional evidence given above, I think he is not likely to do that; unless, indeed, it be that along with readiness to base conclusions on things "it is easy to imagine" there goes reluctance to accept testimony which it is difficult to doubt. Second, he is supposed to reply that "the germ-plasm of the first sire has in some way or another become partly commingled with that of the immature ova"; and Dr. Romanes goes on to describe how there may be millions of spermatozoa and "thousands of millions" of their contained "ids" around the ovaries, to which these secondary effects are due. But, on the one hand, he does not explain why in such case each subsequent ovum, as it becomes matured, is not fertilized by the sperm-cells present, or their contained germ-plasm, rendering all subsequent fecundations needless; and, on the other hand, he does not explain why, if this does not happen, the potency of this remaining germ-plasm is nevertheless such as to affect not only the next succeeding offspring, but all subsequent offspring. The irreconcilability of these two implications would, I think, sufficiently dispose of the supposition, even had we not daily multitudinous proof that the surface of a mammalian ovarium is not a sperm-atheca. The third difficulty Dr. Romanes urges is the inconceivability of the process by which the germ-plasm of a preceding male parent affects the constitution of the female and her subsequent offspring. In response, I have to ask why he piles up a mountain of difficulties based on the assumption that Mr. Darwin's explanation of heredity by "Pangenesis" is the only available explanation preceding that of Weismann? and why he presents these difficulties to me more especially, deliberately ignoring my own hypothesis of physiological units? It cannot be that he is ignorant of this hypothesis, since the work in which it is variously set forth ("Principles of Biology," §§ 66-97) is one with which he is well acquainted: witness his "Scientific Evidences of Organic Evolution"; and he has had recent reminders of it in Weismann's "Germ-plasm," where it is repeatedly referred to. Why, then, does he assume that I abandon my own hypothesis and adopt that of Darwin, thereby entangling myself in difficulties which my own hypothesis avoids? If, as I have argued, the germ-plasm consists of substantially similar units (having only those minute differences expressive of individual and ancestral differences of structure), none of the complicated requirements which Dr. Romanes emphasises exists, and the alleged inconceivability disappears.

To this I responded, in the *Contemporary Review* for June:—

With regard to the influence of a previous sire, I ventured in my article to show that, even supposing it to be a fact, the phenomena concerned would not constitute any valid evidence against Weismann's theory of germ-plasm, and, of course, still less would "they prove that while the reproductive cells multiply and arrange themselves during the evolution of the embryo, some of their germ-plasm passes into the mass of somatic cells constituting the parental body, and becomes a permanent component of it," with the result that the phenomena in question "are simply fatal to Weismann's hypothesis." For a much simpler and more probable explanation is to be found in supposing that the unused germ-plasm of the first sire may survive the disintegration of its containing spermatozoa in the Fallopian tubes of the female, and thus gain access to the hitherto unripe ova *directly*, instead of first having to affect the whole maternal organism, and then being *reflected* from it to them. I showed, at some length, how immensely complex the mechanism of any such process would necessarily have to be; and for the purposes of exposition I employed the terminology of Darwin's theory of Pangenesis. Mr. Spencer now says: "In response, I have to ask why he [I] piles up a mountain of difficulties based on the assumption that Mr. Darwin's explanation of heredity by 'Pangenesis' is the only available explanation preceding that of Weismann? and why he presents these difficulties to me more expecially, deliberately ignoring my own hypothesis of physiological units?" Now my answer to this is very simple. I do not hold a brief for Weismann. On the contrary, I am in large measure an opponent of his views, and my only object in publishing my previous article was to save the theory of use-inheritance from what seemed to me the weaker parts of Mr. Spencer's advocacy, while thus all the more emphasizing my acceptance of its stronger parts. Therefore, the impression which he seems to have gained from my attempts at impartiality is entirely erroneous. Far from "deliberately ignoring" any of his arguments or hypotheses which seemed to me at all available on the side of use-inheritance, I everywhere endeavoured to make the most of them. And, as regards this particular instance, I expressly used the term "gemmules," instead of "physiological units," simply because I could not see that, as far as my "mountain of difficulties" was concerned, it could make one atom of difference which term I employed. It now appears, however, that, in Mr. Spencer's opinion, there is some very great difference. For, while he allows that the "mountain of difficulties" which I have "piled up" against his interpretation of the alleged phenomena would be valid on the supposition that the ultimate carriers of heredity are "gemmules," he denies that such is the case if we suppose these ultimate carriers to be "physiological units." For this statement, however, he gives no justification; and, as I am unable to conceive wherein the difference lies, I sincerely hope that in any subsequent editions of his pamphlet Mr. Spencer will furnish the requisite explanation. Gladly substituting the words "physiological units" wherever I have used the word "gemmules," I am genuinely anxious to ascertain how he would overcome the "mountain of difficulties" in question. For I do not regard the subject as one of mere dialectics. It is a subject of no small importance to the general issue, Weismann *versus* Lamarck; and, therefore, if Mr. Spencer could show that the phenomena in question make exclusively in favour of the latter, as he alleges, he might profitably inform us in what way he supposes them to do so.

In conclusion, I would like to take this opportunity of explaining that my former article was written in Madeira, where I did not receive a copy of Weismann's most recent work, entitled *The Germ-plasm*, until the *Contemporary Review* for April was being printed off. Thus, I was not then aware that in this work Professor Weismann had fully anticipated several of Mr. Spencer's criticisms—including this matter of the influence of a previous sire. Here he adopts exactly the position which in my article I surmised that he would; so that, to all who have read *The Germ-plasm*, it must have appeared that I was prophesying after the event. Hence the need of this explanation.

Lastly, in the same issue of the *Contemporary Review*, Mr. Spencer explained:—

> Mr. Darwin's hypothesis of Pangenesis implies not only that the reproductive cell must contain numerous kinds of gemmules derived from different organs, but that the numbers of these gemmules must bear to one another something like the proportions which the originating organs bear to one another in size. The conception involves many different *kinds*, whose numbers are in many different *proportions*, and I supposed the difficulty alleged was, that for the influence of a previous sire to be communicated from the growing fœtus to the mother would imply not only the transfer of the various kinds of gemmules derived from him, but also maintenance of their numerical proportions, and that again these gemmules, diffused throughout the maternal system, would have to be transferred in these proportions to the subsequently formed ova. No such difficulties arise if the units conveying hereditary characters are of one kind only.

From this it is apparent that Mr. Spencer has misunderstood "the difficulty alleged," and that the desired explanation is not yet forthcoming. I did not say anything about "kinds" or "proportions" of the carriers of heredity; my difficulty is to conceive of any mechanism whereby these carriers can first directly influence the somatic-cells of the mother, and then indirectly reflect this influence upon her germ-cells. Also, I cannot see any obvious necessity for the intervention of the "embryo" in the process.

www.ingramcontent.com/pod-product-compliance
Lightning Source LLC
Chambersburg PA
CBHW070909180526
45168CB00005B/1986